A Bone to Pick

Also by Mark Bittman

Mark Bittman
A Bone to Pick

The Good and Bad News about Food,

with Wisdom, Insights, and

Advice on Diets, Food Safety, GMOs,

Farming, and More

|>|<

PAM KRAUSS BOOKS

New York

Published in the United States by Pam Krauss Books,
an imprint of the Crown Publishing Group, a division of
Penguin Random House LLC, New York.

www.crownpublishing.com
www.clarksonpotter.com

PAM KRAUSS BOOKS and colophon are trademarks of
Penguin Random House LLC.

All the essays contained in this work were originally
published in the *New York Times* opinion column between
February 2011 and June 2014.

Library of Congress Cataloging-in-Publication Data
Bittman, Mark.
[Essays. Selections]
A bone to pick : the good and bad news about food, with
wisdom, insights, and advice on diets, food safety, GMOs,
farming, and more / Mark Bittman.
pages   cm
Collection of articles published in the *New York Times*.
Includes index.
1. Food industry and trade—United States. 2. Agriculture
and state—United States. 3. Nutrition policy—United
States. 4. Diet—United States. I. Title.
HD9000.9.U5B48 2015
338.10973—dc23
2014044874

ISBN 978-0-8041-8654-4
eBook ISBN 978-0-8041-8655-1

Printed in the United States
Book design by Laura Palese
Jacket design by Kelly Doe
Front jacket photographs by Siede Preis/Getty Images
(pitchfork); Ryan McVay/Getty Images (fork)

10 9 8 7 6 5 4 3 2 1

First Edition

Dedicated to Murray Bittman, 1923–2014

Contents

1 Big Ag, Sustainability, and What's in Between

2 What's Wrong with Meat?

3 What Is Food? And What Is Not?

4 The Truth About Diet(s)

5 The Broken Food Chain

Introduction

America's food system is broken.

Ten years ago, that statement would have been met with blank stares: Most of us didn't know exactly what a "food system" was, let alone that ours wasn't working: after all, we have an affordable, abundant, and mostly safe food supply. But as issues of how our food is produced and consumed, and the impact of both on our health and the environment, have crept further into mainstream culture, media, and politics, more of us are realizing what's at stake, and are joining the conversation. And when it comes to recognizing, assessing, and fixing the shortcomings of our food system, there is a whole lot to talk about.

What you'll find in the following pages is drawn from the writings I have contributed to that conversation. All of it comes from the *New York Times*, mostly from my weekly opinion column, the rest from the *Sunday Magazine*. These articles explore a range of topics as vast and varied as food itself: agriculture, environment, labor, legislation, health, hunger, diet, cooking, food safety, and more.

Taken together in this way the columns form a kind of mosaic, one that's tiled with problems and solutions alike. The problems are numerous and complex, and these are just some of them: Our fossil fuel- and chemical-dependent system of agriculture robs the land of resources in the name of feeding the world. At least a billion people globally—including many millions of Americans—still go hungry. Animals are mass-produced and effectively tortured, and food system workers don't have it good, either. The standard American diet—too much meat, sugar, and hyperprocessed junk—is fueling an astronomically expensive epidemic of preventable lifestyle diseases for which we are all paying. And to top it all off, the politicians who hold the most power for positive change are all too often in the pockets of special interests that fight and spend to preserve the status quo.

Solving these problems requires the kinds of sweeping changes that are only possible through collective action, consciousness-raising, rabble-rousing, and political reform; voting out the bad and electing the good is only a part of the solution. We need activists on all levels, people doing the right thing independently of government, and that goes from cooking regularly to making sure school lunches aren't poison to labor organizing to supporting farmers.

Following you'll find my first column for the *Times* Opinion section. Though now four years old, it remains as good a summary of the current domestic situation as I could muster then, or now. But as I write this—just after Election Day 2014—there are reasons to be both optimistic (Berkeley has passed a soda tax; the school lunch program is better than ever; food workers lead the fight for a better minimum wage) and pessimistic (the Farm Bill is as bad as ever; clean water and air and food safety are all under attack; antibiotics are still used routinely in raising animals). But one thing is certain: There is plenty of good work to do.

I'm lucky and privileged to have a platform from which I can say these things, and hope you find reading this collection as inspiring and energizing as I have found the writing of it.

—MARK BITTMAN
NEW YORK, FALL 2014

A Food Manifesto for the Future

For decades, Americans believed that we had the world's healthiest and safest diet. We worried little about this diet's effect on the environment or on the lives of the animals (or even the workers) it relies upon. Nor did we worry about its ability to endure—that is, its sustainability.

That didn't mean all was well. And we've come to recognize that our diet is unhealthful and unsafe. Many food production workers labor in difficult, even deplorable, conditions, and animals are produced as if they were widgets. It would be hard to devise a more wasteful, damaging, unsustainable system.

Here are some ideas—frequently discussed, but sadly not yet implemented— that would make the growing, preparation, and consumption of food healthier, saner, more productive, less damaging, and more enduring. In no particular order:

- End government subsidies to processed food. We grow more corn for livestock and cars than for humans, and it's subsidized by more than $3 billion annually; most of it is processed beyond recognition. The story is similar for other crops, including soy: 98 percent of soybean meal becomes livestock feed, while most soybean oil is used in processed foods. Meanwhile, the marketers of the junk food made from these crops receive tax write-offs for the costs of promoting their wares. Total agricultural subsidies in 2009 were around $16 billion, which would pay for a great many of the ideas that follow.

- Begin subsidies to those who produce and sell actual food for direct consumption. Small farmers and their employees need to make living wages. Markets—from super- to farmers'—should be supported when they open in so-called food deserts and when they focus on real food rather than junk food. And, of course, we should immediately increase subsidies for school lunches so we can feed our youth more real food.

- Break up the U.S. Department of Agriculture and empower the Food and Drug Administration. Currently, the U.S.D.A. counts among its missions both expanding markets for agricultural products (like corn and soy!) and providing nutrition education. These goals are at odds with each other; you can't sell garbage while telling people not to eat it, and we need an agency devoted to encouraging sane eating. Meanwhile, the F.D.A. must be given expanded powers to ensure the safety of our food supply. (Food-related deaths are far more common than those resulting from terrorism, yet the F.D.A.'s budget is about one-fifteenth that of Homeland Security.)

- Outlaw concentrated animal feeding operations and encourage the development of sustainable animal husbandry. The concentrated system degrades the environment, directly and indirectly, while torturing animals and producing tainted meat, poultry, eggs, and, more recently, fish. Sustainable methods of producing meat for consumption exist. At the same time, we must educate and encourage Americans to eat differently. It's difficult to find a principled nutrition and health expert who doesn't believe that a largely plant-based diet is the way to promote health and attack chronic diseases, which are now bigger killers, worldwide, than communicable ones. Furthermore, plant-based diets ease environmental stress, including global warming.

- Encourage and subsidize home cooking. (Someday soon, I'll write about my idea for a new Civilian Cooking Corps.) When people cook their own food, they make better choices. When families eat together, they're more stable. We should provide food education for children (a new form of home ec, anyone?), cooking classes for anyone who wants them, and even cooking assistance for those unable to cook for themselves.

- Tax the marketing and sale of unhealthful foods. Another budget booster. This isn't nanny-state paternalism but an accepted role of government: public health. If you support seat-belt, tobacco, and al-cohol laws, sewer systems and traffic lights, you should support leg-islation curbing the relentless marketing of soda and other foods that are hazardous to our health—including the sacred cheeseburger and fries.

- Reduce waste and encourage recycling. The environmental stress incurred by unabsorbed fertilizer cannot be overestimated, and has caused, for example, a 6,000-square-mile dead zone in the Gulf of Mexico that is probably more damaging than the BP oil spill. And some estimates indicate that we waste half the food that's grown. A careful look at ways to reduce waste and promote recycling is in order.

- Mandate truth in labeling. Nearly everything labeled "healthy" or "natural" is not. It's probably too much to ask that "vitamin water" be called "sugar water with vitamins," but that's precisely what real truth in labeling would mean.

- Reinvest in research geared toward leading a global movement in sus-tainable agriculture, combining technology and tradition to create a new and meaningful Green Revolution.

The essential message is this: food and everything surrounding it is a cru-cial matter of personal and public health, of national and global security. At stake is not only the health of humans but that of the earth.

FEBRUARY 2, 2011

Big Ag, Sustainability, and What's in Between

You can eat without farms, but for the last 10,000 years few humans have. For about 9,900 of those years, though, all farms were small and—at least arguably—more or less sustainable. That is, they put back into the earth, in the form of animal and even human waste and plant matter, just about as much as they took out. There were no synthetic fertilizers, pesticides, and so on, and everything was pretty much what we'd now call organic.

Much has changed. The dominant form of agriculture in the West is industrial, large-scale, fossil fuel and chemical dependent, and heavy on water use. It isn't sustainable—that is, it uses far more in resources than it returns to the land—and it poisons land, sea, animals, workers, and consumers. It's used primarily to grow a half dozen crops, among them corn and soybeans, much of which, sadly, are fed to animals, used as fuel (ethanol), or converted into the kind of junk that's largely responsible for obesity. And despite the fact that there's enough food produced to feed everyone on the planet adequately, tens of millions of Americans, and more than a billion people worldwide, struggle with hunger.

In short, it's a terrible "system," and one that could be improved almost immeasurably if just a little bit of care were taken.

How to Feed the World

I t's been 50 years since President John F. Kennedy spoke of ending world hunger, yet on the eve of World Food Day, Oct. 16, the situation remains dire. The question "How will we feed the world?" implies that we have no choice but to intensify industrial agriculture, with more high-tech seeds, chemicals, and collateral damage. Yet there are other, better options.

Something approaching a billion people are hungry, a number that's been fairly stable for more than 50 years, although it has declined as a percentage of the total population.

"Feeding the world" might as well be a marketing slogan for Big Ag, a euphemism for "Let's ramp up sales," as if producing more cars would guarantee that everyone had one. But if it worked that way, surely the rate of hunger in the United States would not be the highest percentage of any developed nation, a rate closer to that of Indonesia than of Britain.

The world has long produced enough calories, around 2,700 per day per human, more than enough to meet the United Nations projection of a population of nine billion in 2050, up from the current seven billion. There are hungry people not because food is lacking, but because not all of those calories go to feed humans (a third go to feed animals, nearly 5 percent are used to produce biofuels, and as much as a third is wasted, all along the food chain).

The current system is neither environmentally nor economically sustainable, dependent as it is on fossil fuels and routinely resulting in environmental damage. It's geared to letting the half of the planet with money eat well while everyone else scrambles to eat as cheaply as possible.

While a billion people are hungry, about three billion people are not eating well, according to the United Nations Food and Agriculture Organization, if you count obese and overweight people alongside those with micronutrient deficiencies. Paradoxically, as increasing numbers of people can afford to eat well, food for the poor will become scarcer, because demand for animal products will surge, and they require more resources like grain to produce. A global population growth of less than 30 percent is projected to double the demand for animal products. But there is not the land, water, or fertilizer—let alone the health care funding—for the world to consume Western levels of meat.

If we want to ensure that poor people eat and also do a better job than "modern" farming does at preserving the earth's health and productivity, we must stop assuming that the industrial model of food production and its accompanying disease-producing diet is both inevitable and desirable. I have dozens of friends and colleagues who say things like, "I hate industrial ag, but how will we feed the poor?"

Let's at last recognize that there are two food systems, one industrial and one of small landholders, or peasants if you prefer. The peasant system is not only here for good, it's arguably more efficient than the industrial model. According to the ETC Group, a research and advocacy organization based in Ottawa, the industrial food chain uses 70 percent of agricultural resources to provide 30 percent of the world's food, whereas what ETC calls "the peasant food web" produces the remaining 70 percent using only 30 percent of the resources.

Yes, it is true that high-yielding varieties of any major commercial monoculture crop will produce more per acre than peasant-bred varieties of the same crop. But by diversifying crops, mixing plants and animals, planting trees— which provide not only fruit but shelter for birds, shade, fertility through nutrient recycling, and more—small landholders can produce more food (and more kinds of food) with fewer resources and lower transportation costs (which means a lower carbon footprint), while providing greater food security, maintaining greater biodiversity, and even better withstanding the effects of climate change. (Not only that: their techniques have been demonstrated to be effective on larger-scale farms, even in the Corn Belt of the United States.) And all of this without the level of subsidies and other support that industrial agriculture has received in the last half-century, and despite the efforts of Big Ag to become even more dominant.

In fact if you define "productivity" not as pounds per acre but as the number of people fed per that same area, you find that the United States ranks behind both China and India (and indeed the world average), and roughly the same as Bangladesh, because so much of what we grow goes to animals and biofuels.

(Regardless of how food is produced, delivered, and consumed, waste remains at about one third.) Thus, as the ETC's research director, Kathy Jo Wetter, says, "It would be lunacy to hold that the current production paradigm based on multinational agribusiness is the only credible starting point for achieving food security." This is especially true given all of its downsides.

As Raj Patel, a fellow at the Institute for Food and Development Policy, puts it, "The playing field has been tilted against peasants for centuries, and they've still managed to feed more people than industrial agriculture. With the right kinds of agroecological training and the freedom to shape the food system on fair terms, it's a safe bet that they'll be able to feed themselves, and others as well."

Yet obviously not all poor people feed themselves well, because they lack the essentials: land, water, energy, and nutrients. Often that's a result of cruel dictatorship (North Korea) or war, displacement and strife (the Horn of Africa, Haiti, and many other places), or drought or other calamities. But it can also be an intentional and direct result of land and food speculation and land and water grabs, which make it impossible for peasants to remain in their home villages. (Governments of many developing countries may also act as agents for industrial agriculture, seeing peasant farming as "inefficient.")

The result is forced flight to cities, where peasants become poorly paid laborers, enter the cash market for (increasingly mass produced) food, and eat worse. (They're no longer "peasants," at this point, but more akin to the working poor of the United States, who also often cannot afford to eat well, though not to the point of starvation.) It's a formula for making not only hunger but obesity: remove the ability to produce food, then remove the ability to pay for food, or replace it with only one choice: bad food.

It's not news that the poor need money and justice. If there's a bright side here, it's that the changes required to "fix" the problems created by "industrial agriculture" are perhaps more tractable than those created by inequality.

We might begin by ditching the narrow focus on yields (as Jonathan Foley, director of the Institute on the Environment at the University of Minnesota, says, "It's not 'grow baby grow'"), which seem to be ebbing naturally as land quality deteriorates and chemicals become less effective (despite high-tech "advances" like genetically engineered crops). Better, it would seem, would be to ask not how much food is produced, but how it's produced, for whom, at what price, cost, and benefit.

We also need to see more investment in researching the benefits of traditional farming. Even though simple techniques like those mentioned above give measurably excellent results, because they're traditional—even ancient— "technologies," and because their benefits in profiting multinationals or international trade are limited, they've never received investment on the same scale as corporate agriculture. (It's impossible not to point out here that a similar situation exists between highly subsidized and damaging fossil fuels and oft-ignored yet environmentally friendly renewables.)

Instead, the money and energy (of all kinds) focused on boosting supply cannot be overstated. If equal resources were put into reducing waste—which aside from its obvious merits would vastly prevent the corresponding greenhouse gas emissions—questioning the value of animal products, reducing overconsumption (where "waste" becomes "waist"), actively promoting saner, less energy-consuming alternatives, and granting that peasants have the right to farm their traditional landholdings, we could not only ensure that people could feed themselves but also reduce agriculture's contribution to greenhouse gases, chronic disease, and energy depletion.

This isn't about "organic" versus "modern." It's about supporting the system in which small producers make decisions based on their knowledge and experience of their farms in the landscape, as opposed to buying standardized technological fixes in a bag. Some people call this knowledge-based rather than energy-based agriculture, but obviously it takes plenty of energy; as it happens, much of that energy is human, which can be a good thing. Frances Moore Lappé, author of *Diet for a Small Planet,* calls it "relational," and says, "Agroecology is not just healthy sustainable food production but the seed of a different way of relating to one another, and to the earth."

That may sound new age-y, but so be it; all kinds of questions and all kinds of theories are needed if we're going to produce food sustainably. Supporting, or at least not obstructing, peasant farming is one key factor, but the other is reining in Western-style monoculture and the standard American diet it creates.

Some experts are at least marginally optimistic about the second half of this: "The trick is to find the sweet spot," says Mr. Foley of the University of Minnesota, "between better nutrition and eating too much meat and junk. The optimistic view is to hope that the conversation about what's wrong with our diet may deflect some of this. Eating more meat is voluntary, and how the Chinese middle class winds up eating will determine a great deal." Of course, at the moment, that middle class shows every indication that it's moving in the wrong direction; China is the world's leading consumer of meat, a trend that isn't slowing.

But if the standard American diet represents the low point of eating, a question is whether the developing world, as it hurtles toward that nutritional nadir—the polar opposite of hunger, but almost as deadly—can see its destructive nature and pull out of the dive before its diet crashes. Because "solving" hunger by driving people into cities to take low-paying jobs so they can buy burgers and fries is hardly a desirable outcome.

OCTOBER 14, 2013

Sustainable Farming Can Feed the World

The oldest and most common dig against organic agriculture is that it cannot feed the world's citizens; this, however, is a supposition, not a fact. And industrial agriculture isn't working perfectly, either: the global food price index is at a record high, and our agricultural system is wreaking havoc with the health not only of humans but of the earth. There are around a billion undernourished people; we can also thank the current system for the billion who are overweight or obese.

Yet there is good news: increasing numbers of scientists, policy panels, and experts (not hippies!) are suggesting that agricultural practices pretty close to organic—perhaps best called "sustainable"—can feed more poor people sooner, begin to repair the damage caused by industrial production, and, in the long term, become the norm.

Olivier de Schutter, the United Nations' special rapporteur on the Right to Food, is the author of a report entitled "Agro-ecology and the Right to Food." (Agro-ecology, he explained to me, has "lots" in common with both "sustainable" and "organic.") Chief among de Schutter's recommendations is this: "Agriculture should be fundamentally redirected towards modes of production that are more environmentally sustainable and socially just." Agro-ecology, he said, immediately helps "small farmers who must be able to farm in ways that are less expensive and more productive. But it benefits all of us, because it decelerates global warming and ecological destruction." Further, by decentralizing production, floods in Southeast Asia, for example, might not mean huge shortfalls in the world's rice crop; smaller scale farming makes the system less susceptible to climate shocks. (Calling it a system is a convention; it's actually quite anarchic, what with all these starving and overweight people canceling each other out.)

Industrial (or "conventional," even though by most standards it's anything but) agriculture requires a great deal of resources, including disproportionate amounts of water and the fossil fuel that's needed for transportation, to make chemical fertilizer, mechanize working the land and its crops, run irrigation sources, and heat buildings and crop dryers. This means it needs more in the way of resources than the earth can replenish. (Fun/depressing fact: It takes the earth 18 months to replenish the amount of resources we use each year. Looked at another way, we'd need 1.5 earths to be sustainable at our current rate of consumption.)

Agro-ecology and related methods are going to require resources too, but they're more in the form of labor, both intellectual—much research remains to be done—and physical: the world will need more farmers, and quite possibly less mechanization. Many adherents rule out nothing, including in their recommendations even GMOs and chemical fertilizers where justifiable. Meanwhile, those working towards improving conventional agriculture are borrowing more from organic methods.

Currently, however, it's difficult to see progress in a country where, for example, nearly 90 percent of the corn crop is used for either ethanol (40 percent) or animal feed (50 percent). And most of the diehard adherents of industrial agriculture—sadly, this usually includes Congress, which largely ignores these issues—act as if we'll somehow "fix" global warming and the resulting climate change. (The small percentage of climate-change deniers are still arguing with Copernicus.) Their assumption is that by increasing supply, we'll eventually figure out how to feed everyone on earth, even though we don't do that now, our population is going to be nine billion by 2050, and more supply of the wrong things—oil, corn, beef—only worsens things. Many seem to naively believe that we won't run out of the resources we need to keep this system going.

There is more than a bit of silver-bullet thinking here. Yet anyone who opens his or her eyes sees a natural world so threatened by industrial agriculture that it's tempting to drop off the grid and raise a few chickens.

To back up and state some obvious goals: We need a global perspective, the (moral) recognition that food is a basic right and the (practical) one that sustainability is a high priority. We want to reduce and repair environmental damage, cut back on the production and consumption of resource-intensive food, increase efficiency, and do something about waste. (Some estimate that

50 percent of all food is wasted.) A sensible and nutritious diet for everyone is essential; many people will eat better, and others may eat fewer animal products, which is also eating better.

De Schutter and others who agree with the goals of the previous paragraph say that sustainable agriculture should be the immediate choice for underdeveloped countries, and that even developed countries should take only the best aspects of conventional agriculture along on a ride that leaves all but the best of its methods behind. Just last month, the U.K.'s government office for science published "The Future of Food and Farming," which is both damning of the current resource-intensive system (though it is decidedly pro-GMO) and encouraging of sustainable, and which led de Schutter to say that studies demonstrate that sustainable agriculture can more than double yields in just a few years.

No one knows how many people can be fed this way, but a number of experts and studies—including those from the U.N. Food and Agriculture Organization, the University of Michigan, and Worldwatch—seem to be lining up to suggest that sustainable agriculture is a system more people should choose. For developing nations, especially those in Africa, the shift from high- to low-tech farming can happen quickly, said de Schutter: "It's easiest to make the transition in places that still have a direction to take." But, he added, although "in developed regions the shift away from industrial mode will be difficult to achieve," ultimately even those countries most "addicted" to chemical fertilizers must change.

"We have to move towards sustainable production," he said. "We cannot depend on the gas fields of Russia or the oil fields of the Middle East, and we cannot continue to destroy the environment and accelerate climate change. We must adopt the most efficient farming techniques available."

And those, he and others emphasize, are not industrial but sustainable.

MARCH 8, 2011

Pesticides: Now More Than Ever

Height how quickly we forget.

After the publication of *Silent Spring*, 50 years ago, we (scientists, environmental and health advocates, birdwatchers, citizens) managed to curb the use of pesticides and our exposure to them—only to see their application grow to the point where American agriculture uses more of them than ever before.

And the threat is more acute than ever. While Rachel Carson focused on their effect on "nature," it's become obvious that farmworkers need protection from direct exposure while applying chemicals to crops. (Cancer, of course, is one awful risk of exposure. But there is the very real danger of anencephaly—a birth defect in which the baby is born without parts of brain and/or skull—in the children of farmworkers, both men and women, who were exposed to pesticides, even before pregnancy.) Less well known are the recent studies showing that routine, casual, continuing—what you might call chronic—exposure to pesticides is damaging not only to flora but to all creatures, including the one that habitually considers itself above it all: us.

I was impressed by a statement by the American Academy of Pediatrics—not exactly a radical organization—warning parents of the dangers of pesticides and recommending that they try to reduce contact with them. The accompanying report calls the evidence "robust" for associations between pesticide exposure and cancer (specifically brain tumors and leukemia) and "adverse" neurodevelopment, including lowered I.Q., autism, and attention disorders and hyperactivity. (Alzheimer's, obviously not a pediatric concern, has also been linked to pesticide exposure.)

This reminded me of recently disclosed evidence showing that pesticide exposure in pregnant women may be obesogenic—that is, it may cause their children to tend to become obese. The mechanism for this is beginning to be understood, and it's not entirely shocking, because many pesticides have been shown to be endocrine disruptors, changing gene expression patterns and causing unforeseen harm to health.

And that in turn prompted me to recall that genetically engineered crops, ostensibly designed in part to reduce the need for pesticides, have—thanks to pesticide-resistant "superweeds"—actually increased our pesticide use steadily over the last decade or so. (In general, fields growing crops using genetically engineered seeds use 24 percent more chemicals than those grown with conventional seeds.)

Although these all caught my attention, the most striking non-event of the last year—decade, generation—is how asleep at the wheel we have all been regarding pesticides. Because every human tested is found to have pesticides in his or her body fat. And because pesticides are found in nearly every stream in the United States, over 90 percent of wells, and—in urban and agricultural areas—over half the groundwater. So Department of Agriculture data show that the average American is exposed to 10 or more pesticides every day, via diet and drinking water.

This shouldn't be surprising: pesticide drift is a term used to describe the phenomenon by which almost all pesticides—95 to 98 percent is the number I've seen—wind up on or in something other than their intended target. (This means, of course, that in order to be effective more pesticides must be used than would be necessary if targeting were more accurate.)

Much damage has been done, and it's going to get worse before it gets better. The long-term solution is to reduce pesticide use, and the ways to do that include some of the typical laundry-list items that find their way into every "how to improve American agriculture" story: rotate crops, which reduces attacks by invasive species; employ integrated pest management, which basically means "think before you spray"; better regulate pesticides (and both increase funding for and eliminate the revolving door policy at the Environmental Protection Agency) with an eye toward protecting the most vulnerable—that is, farmworkers, anyone of childbearing age, and especially women in their first trimester of pregnancy; give farmers options for "conventional," that is, non-genetically engineered seeds (around 95 percent of all seeds for soy, corn, and cotton contain a pesticide-resistant gene, which encourages wanton spraying); and in general move toward using more organic principles.

Note, please, that only this last strategy helps us protect ourselves and our families now. But although there's the usual disclaimer that not everyone can afford organic food, at a time when organic food has been under attack it's important to remember that part of the very reason for its existence is to bring food to the market that, if not free of all traces of pesticides—remember drift—at least contains none that have been applied intentionally. Charles Benbrook, in his excellent 2008 report "Simplifying the Pesticide Risk Equation: The Organic Option," estimates that organic food production would reduce our overall exposure to pesticides by 97 percent; that is, all but eliminate it.

If I were of child-rearing age now, or the parent of young children, I would make every effort to buy organic food. If I couldn't do that, I would rely on the Environmental Working Group's guide to pesticides in produce. (Their "Dirty Dozen" lists those fruits and vegetables with highest pesticide residues, and their "Clean Fifteen" notes those that are lowest.) But regardless of age, we need to stay awake, and remember that the dangers of pesticides are as real now as they were half a century ago.

DECEMBER 11, 2012

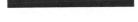

That Flawed Stanford Study

I tried to ignore the "Stanford study." I really did. It made so little sense that I thought it would have little impact.

That was dumb of me, and I'm sorry.

The study, which suggested—incredibly—that there is no "strong evidence that organic foods are significantly more nutritious than conventional foods," caused as great an uproar as anything that has happened, food-wise, this year. (By comparison, the Alzheimer's/diabetes link I covered was virtually ignored.)

That's because headlines (and, of course, tweets) matter. The Stanford study was not only an exercise in misdirection, it was a headline generator. By providing "useful" and "counterintuitive" information about organic food, it played right into the hands of the news hungry while conveniently obscuring important features of organic agriculture.

If I may play with metaphor for a moment, the study was like declaring guns no more dangerous than baseball bats when it comes to blunt-object head injuries. It was the equivalent of comparing milk and Elmer's glue on the basis of whiteness. It did, in short, miss the point. Even Crystal Smith-Spangler, a Stanford coauthor, perfectly captured the narrowness of the study when she said: "some believe that organic food is always healthier and more nutritious. We were a little surprised that we didn't find that." That's because they didn't look—or even worse, they ignored.

In fact, the Stanford study—actually a meta-study, an analysis of more than 200 existing studies—does say that "consumption of organic foods may reduce exposure to pesticide residues and antibiotic-resistant bacteria."

Since that's largely why people eat organic foods, what's the big deal?

Especially if we refer to common definitions of "nutritious" and point out that, in general, nutritious food promotes health and good condition. How can something that reduces your exposure to pesticides and antibiotic-resistant bacteria not be "more nutritious" than food that doesn't?

Because the study narrowly defines "nutritious" as containing more vitamins. Dr. Dena Bravata, the study's senior author, conceded that there are other reasons why people opt for organic (the aforementioned pesticides and bacteria chief among them) but said that if the decision between buying organic or conventional food were based on nutrients, "there is not robust evidence to choose one or the other." By which standard you can claim that, based on nutrients, Frosted Flakes are a better choice than an apple.

But they're not. And overlooking these key factors allows the authors to imply that there isn't "robust" evidence to choose organic food over conventional. (Which for many people there is.) Under the convenient cover of helping consumers make informed choices, the study constructed a set of criteria that would easily allow them to cut "organic" down to size.

Suspect conclusions derived from suspect studies are increasingly common, including these recent examples: having a poor sense of smell might be linked to being a psychopath. People who read food labels are thinner. GMOs give rats tumors. (That one in particular violated many rules of both science and ethics.) Usually these "revelations" are of little more than passing interest, but they can sometimes be downright destructive. Susan Clark, the executive director of the Columbia Foundation, summed up the flaws of the Stanford approach perfectly in a letter to her colleagues:

"The researchers started with a narrow set of assumptions and arrived at entirely predictable conclusions. Stanford should be ashamed of the lack of expertise about food and farming among the researchers, a low level of academic rigor in the study, its biased conclusions, and lack of transparency about the industry ties of the major researchers on the study. Normally we busy people would simply ignore another useless academic study, but this study was so aggressively spun by the PR masters that it requires a response."

When Clark says "aggressively spun by the PR masters," this is what she means: a Google search for "Stanford Annals of Internal Medicine" gave me these six results in the top seven:

Stanford Scientists Cast Doubt on Advantages of Organic Meat and Produce (*New York Times*)

Why Organic Food May Not Be Healthier for You (NPR)

Organic food no more nutritious than non-organic, study finds (MSNBC)

Organic Food Is No Healthier Than Conventional Food (*U.S. News and World Report*)

Study Questions How Much Better Organic Food Is (A.P., via Google)

Save Your Cash? Organic Food Is Not Healthier: Stanford U. (*New York Daily News*)

Yet even within its narrow framework it appears the Stanford study was incorrect. Last year Kirsten Brandt, a researcher from Newcastle University, published a similar analysis of existing studies and wound up with the opposite result, concluding that organic foods are actually more nutritious. In combing through the Stanford study she's not only noticed a critical error in properly identifying a class of nutrients, a spelling error indicative of biochemical incompetence (or at least an egregious oversight) that skewed one important result, but also that the researchers curiously excluded evaluating many nutrients that she found to be considerably higher in organic foods.

Even the website of Stanford's Freeman Spogli Institute for International Studies (which supported the research) features an article right above that about the new study that says "study confirms value of organic farming" and details how conventional agriculture is much more likely to contaminate drinking water with nitrates, which "can cause serious illness in humans, particularly small children." What's healthy and nutritious again?

Like too many studies, the Stanford study dangerously isolates a finding from its larger context. It significantly plays down the disparity in pesticides and neglects to mention that workers get a pesticide-poisoning diagnosis each year. And while the study concedes that "the risk for isolating bacteria resistant to three or more antibiotics was 33 percent higher among conventional chicken and pork than organic alternatives," it apparently didn't seek to explore how consuming antibiotic-resistant bacteria might be considered "non-nutritious." Finally (I think) it turns out that Cargill (the largest privately held company in the United States) provides major financing for Freeman Spogli, and that's inspired a petition to retract the findings.

That the authors of the study chose to focus on a trivial aspect of the organic versus conventional comparison is regrettable. That they published a study that would so obviously be construed as a blanket knock against organic agriculture is willfully misleading and dangerous. That so many leading news agencies fall for this stuff is scary.

Clark is right: this junk science deserves a response. Ignoring it isn't enough. I apologize.

OCTOBER 2, 2012

A Simple Fix for Farming

It's becoming clear that we can grow all the food we need, and profitably, with far fewer chemicals. And I'm not talking about imposing some utopian vision of small organic farms on the world. So-called conventional agriculture can shed much of its chemical use—if it wants to.

This was hammered home once again in what may be the most important agricultural study this year, although it has been largely ignored by the media, two of the leading science journals, and even one of the study's sponsors, the often hapless Department of Agriculture.

The study was done on land owned by Iowa State University called the Marsden Farm. On 22 acres of it, beginning in 2003, researchers set up three plots: one replicated the typical Midwestern cycle of planting corn one year and then soybeans the next, along with its routine mix of chemicals. On another, they planted a three-year cycle that included oats; the third plot added a four-year cycle and alfalfa. The longer rotations also integrated the raising of livestock, whose manure was used as fertilizer.

The results were stunning: The longer rotations produced better yields of both corn and soy, reduced the need for nitrogen fertilizer and herbicides by up to 88 percent, reduced the amounts of toxins in groundwater 200-fold, and didn't reduce profits by a single cent.

In short, there was only upside—and no downside at all—associated with the longer rotations. There was an increase in labor costs, but remember that profits were stable. So this is a matter of paying people for their knowledge and smart work instead of paying chemical companies for poisons. And it's a high-stakes game; according to the Environmental Protection Agency, about five billion pounds of pesticides are used each year in the United States.

No one expects Iowa corn and soybean farmers to turn this thing around tomorrow, but one might at least hope that the U.S.D.A. would trumpet the outcome. The agency declined to comment when I asked about it. One can guess that perhaps no one at the higher levels even knows about it, or that they're afraid to tell Monsanto about agency-supported research that demonstrates a decreased need for chemicals. (A conspiracy theorist might note that the journals *Science* and *Proceedings of the National Academy of Sciences* both turned down the study. It was finally published in *PLOS ONE*; I first read about it on the Union of Concerned Scientists website.)

Debates about how we grow food are usually presented in a simplistic, black-and-white way, conventional versus organic. (The spectrum that includes conventional on one end and organic on the other is not unlike the one that opposes the standard American diet with veganism.) In farming, you have loads of chemicals and disastrous environmental impact against an orthodox, even dogmatic method that is difficult to carry out on a large scale.

But seeing organic as the only alternative to industrial agriculture, or veganism as the only alternative to supersize me, is a bit like saying that the only alternative to the ravages of capitalism is Stalinism; there are other ways. And positioning organic as the only alternative allows its opponents to point to its flaws and say, "See? We have to remain with conventional."

The Marsden Farm study points to a third path. And though critics of this path can be predictably counted on to say it's moving backward, the increased yields, markedly decreased input of chemicals, reduced energy costs, and stable profits tell another story, one of serious progress.

Nor was this a rinky-dink study: the background and scientific rigor of the authors—who represent the U.S.D.A.'s Agricultural Research Service as well as two of the country's leading agricultural universities—are unimpeachable. When I asked Adam Davis, an author of the study who works for the U.S.D.A., to summarize the findings, he said, "These were simple changes patterned after those used by North American farmers for generations. What we found was that if you don't hold the natural forces back they are going to work for you."

This means that not only is weed suppression a direct result of systematic and increased crop rotation along with mulching, cultivation, and other non-chemical techniques, but that by not poisoning the fields, we make it possible for insects, rodents, and other critters to do their part and eat weeds and their seeds. In addition, by growing forage crops for cattle or other ruminants you can raise healthy animals that not only contribute to the health of the fields but provide fertilizer. (The same manure that's a benefit in a system like this is a pollutant in large-scale, confined animal-rearing operations, where thousands of animals make manure disposal an extreme challenge.)

Perhaps most difficult to quantify is that this kind of farming—more thoughtful and less reflexive—requires more walking of the fields, more observations, more applications of fertilizer and chemicals if, when, and where they're needed, rather than on an all-inclusive schedule. "You substitute producer knowledge for blindly using inputs," Davis says.

So: combine crop rotation, the re-integration of animals into crop production, and intelligent farming, and you can use chemicals (to paraphrase the report's abstract) to fine-tune rather than drive the system, with no loss in performance and in fact the gain of animal products.

Why wouldn't a farmer go this route? One answer is that first he or she has to hear about it. Another, says Matt Liebman, one of the authors of the study and an agronomy professor at Iowa State, is that, "There's no cost assigned to environmental externalities"—the environmental damage done by industrial farming, analogous to the health damage done by the "cheap" standard American diet—"and the profitability of doing things with lots of chemical input isn't questioned."

This study not only questions those assumptions, it demonstrates that the chemicals contributing to "environmental externalities" can be drastically reduced at no sacrifice, except to that of the bottom line of chemical companies. That direction is in the interest of most of us—or at least those whose well-being doesn't rely on that bottom line.

Sadly, it seems there isn't a government agency up to the task of encouraging things to move that way, even in the face of convincing evidence.

OCTOBER 19, 2012

Not All Industrial Food Is Evil

I've long wondered how producing a decent ingredient, one that you can buy in any supermarket, really happens. Take canned tomatoes, of which I probably use 100 pounds a year. It costs $2 to $3 a pound to buy hard, tasteless, "fresh" plum tomatoes, but only half that for almost two pounds of canned tomatoes that taste much better. How is that possible?

The answer lies in a process that is almost unimaginable in scope without seeing it firsthand. So, fearing the worst—because we all "know" that organic farming is "good" and industrial farming is "bad"—I headed to the Sacramento Valley in California to see a big tomato operation.

I began by touring Bruce Rominger's farm in Winters. With his brother Rick and as many as 40 employees, Rominger farms around 6,000 acres of tomatoes, wheat, sunflowers, safflower, onions, alfalfa, sheep, rice, and more. Unlike many Midwestern farm operations, which grow corn and soy exclusively, here are diversity, crop rotation, cover crops, and, for the most part, real food—not crops destined for junk food, animal feed, or biofuel. That's a good start.

On an 82-acre field, tomato plants covered the ground for a hundred yards in every direction. Water and fertilizer are supplied through subsoil irrigation—a network of buried tubing—which reduces waste and runoff and assures roughly uniform delivery along the row. (In older, furrow-irrigated fields—in which ditches next to the rows of plants are flooded with water from a central canal—tomatoes at the ends of rows suffer.)

The tomatoes are bred to ripen simultaneously because there is just one harvest. They're also blocky in shape, the better to move along conveyor belts. Hundreds of types of tomatoes are grown for processing, bred for acidity, disease resistance, use, sweetness, wall thickness, ripening date, and so on. They're not referred to by cuddly names like "Early Girl" but by number: "BQ 205."

I tasted two; they had a firm, pleasant texture and mild but real flavor, and were better than any tomatoes—even so-called heirlooms—sold in my supermarket.

I mounted the harvester, a 35-foot-long machine that cuts the vine underground and lifts it into its belly, where belts and sensors return dirt, vine, root, and green tomatoes to the soil. (All this material is either turned back into the soil or left for sheep to graze on.) Two people on each side sort the continual stream of tomatoes manually before a conveyor transfers the tomatoes by chute to a gondola. When one gondola is full (it holds 25 tons), it's replaced by another. This way, Rominger can harvest around 20 acres in a 24-hour period: 1,000 tons. He estimates his cost at $3,000 per acre and hopes for a $500 profit on each. "Of course," he told me, "sometimes I have a field that collapses on me, and I lose $500."

Fifty years ago, tomatoes were picked by hand, backbreaking piecework that involved filling and lugging 50-pound boxes. Workers had few rights and suffered much abuse, as did the land: irrigation and fertilizer use were more wasteful, and chemicals were applied liberally and by the calendar, not sparingly by need.

Although the mechanical harvester was controversial when it was first introduced—the United Farm Workers fought its use, fearing it would cost jobs—it revolutionized the industry. (Its impact has been compared to that of the cotton gin.) Yields have more than doubled since the 1960s, and California now produces almost all the canned tomatoes and paste in the United States and more than a third of the world's. For 12 to 14 weeks every summer, Rominger and other growers are harvesting 24/7.

The canneries also operate nonstop. My next visit was to Pacific Coast Producers (P.C.P.), a co-op down the road. It packs for Walmart, Safeway, Kroger, Ralphs, and other major chains. Its annual sales—on 20 million cases of whole, diced, crushed, ground, and sliced tomatoes, sauce, paste, and more—are more than $250 million.

Imagine all the tomatoes you've ever seen, multiplied by a thousand, and you begin to get some idea of the lineup outside P.C.P., which in a 24-hour period may go through 300 gondolas, holding 7,500 tons all together.

At P.C.P., workers first random-sample the tomatoes in an elaborate process that determines both where on the processing line the tomatoes wind up (an algorithm decides which fruit from which gondolas to combine for the best-tasting sauce, for example) and the exact amount the growers are paid for that load. This year, it's somewhere around 3.5 cents per pound; if you're wondering what percentage of the price of the canned tomato you buy goes to the farmer, I'm figuring it's around 2.

The cannery itself is a whirlwind of moist, intense heat and subway-level noise. At peak times, P.C.P. employs more than 1,000 workers. My liberal heart was bleeding at the thought of minimum wage for this tough work—some (not all) of these workstations are as unpleasant as any I've seen—but the plant is unionized. So, according to a P.C.P. spokesman, the average wage is about $17 an hour, and there are benefits.

It's far from paradise, but it isn't hell either. The basic question is this: Are the processes and products healthy, fair, green, and affordable?

Workers in the fields have shade, water, and breaks; they're not being paid by the piece. Workers in the plants are not getting rich but they're doing better than they would working in the fields, or in a fast-food joint.

Rominger is managing his fields conscientiously and, by today's standards, progressively. He's also juggling an almost unimaginable array of standards set by the state, by P.C.P. and other processors, and even by his customers, who may say things like, "What are you doing about nitrate runoff?"

The canner P.C.P. is running what appear to be safe and clean production lines while producing close-to-"natural" tomato products that nearly anyone can afford.

Oddly, affordability is not the problem; in fact, the tomatoes are too cheap. If they cost more, farmers like Rominger would be more inclined to grow tomatoes organically; to pay his workers better or offer benefits to more of them; to make a better living himself.

But the processed tomato market is international, with increasing pressure from Italy, China, and Mexico. California has advantages, but it still must compete on price. Producers also compete with one another, making it tough for even the most principled ones to increase worker pay. To see change, then, all workers, globally, must be paid better, so that the price of tomatoes goes up across the board.

How does this happen? Unionization, or an increase in the minimum wage, or both. No one would argue that canned tomatoes should be too expensive for poor people, but by increasing minimum wage in the fields and elsewhere, we raise standards of living and increase purchasing power.

The issue is paying enough for food so that everything involved in producing it—land, water, energy, and labor—is treated well. And since sustainability is a journey, progress is essential. It would be foolish to assert that we're anywhere near the destination, but there is progress—even in those areas appropriately called "industrial."

AUGUST 17, 2013

Local Food: No Elitist Plot

I'm not a jingoist, but I'd prefer that more of my food came from America. It'd be even better, really, if most of it came from within a few hundred miles of where we live. We'd be more secure and better served, and our land would be better used. And I'd feel prouder, as if we had a food culture rather than a food fetish.

The Farm Bill needs to address this issue head-on. But by subsidizing commodities, the existing bill (and food policy in general) pushes things in precisely the opposite direction. (NB: A new bill was signed in 2014; it is not radically different, and is better in some minor ways, worse in others.) The vast majority of our farmland grows corn (we're the world's largest producer), soy, and wheat, and these, along with meat and dairy, make us net exporters of foodstuffs.

Incredibly, however, we are net importers of fruits and vegetables, foods that our land is capable of growing in abundance and once did. Most of our imports are from Mexico, Chile, and Canada, but fresh fruits and especially vegetables are shipped here from all over the world, with significant quantities coming from as far away as India, China, and Thailand. And those imports are growing.

This is just plain embarrassing. Global trade is the norm, but for a country that likes to think of itself as the world's leader in agriculture, to be unable to supply its own fruits and vegetables is pathetic. An older (2007) but likely still valid U.S.D.A. report showed that if Americans were to meet the dietary recommendations for fruit and vegetables, we'd need to more than double our fruit and vegetable acreage. (We also must avoid the Santa Barbara syndrome. There, in one of our top fruit- and vegetable-producing counties, as much food is shipped in as is shipped out, and nearly half the people have trouble affording food.) Of course we grow enough corn to feed not only us but many of the world's hungry (it is a whole grain, after all, when it's minimally processed), but the majority of that corn is fed to animals and automobiles, and almost all of the rest produces junk food.

What's wrong with this picture? The notion of importing fruits and vegetables, the idea of having everything "fresh" all the time, was until recently inconceivable and is likely to become so again, as production and transportation costs rise and the absurdity of the "system" becomes evident even to those who now profit from it. When we ignore large-scale production of local food we invite apocalypse, or at least food shortages.

By creating a perverted norm, in which everything is always everywhere and little is seasonal, we have ceased to rely upon staples: long-keeping foods like grains, beans, and root vegetables, foods that provide nutrition when summer greens, fruits, and vegetables aren't readily available. We expect a steady supply of "fresh" Peruvian asparagus, Canadian tomatoes, South African apples, Dutch peppers, and Mexican broccoli. Those who believe they're entitled to eat any food any time seem to think that predominantly local agriculture is an elitist plot to "force" a more limited diet upon us.

But there's something far more important to fear: that when imports stop we won't have the food to replace them, nor the farmers to grow that food. Besides, how limited was the old-fashioned diet of long-keeping fruits and vegetables (I can think of 20 in a few seconds), preserves like jams and sauerkraut (and kimchi!), and smoked or salted meats? Make that contemporary with the addition of those regional and national foods we freeze or can—every vegetable you can think of, many if not most fruits, a great deal of meat and fish—and you have essentially the diet you're eating now. It may not be perfectly "fresh," but it could be at least semi-local.

This kind of approach—grow what you can close to where you live and eat what you can grow—is obviously nothing new. (Even in my lifetime, I can remember seeing asparagus only in late spring, Macintosh apples in the fall, and Empire apples—long keepers—through the winter.) What's new is the lack of farmland, because much has been lost to sprawl or commodity crops, and farmers who can make it happen, farmers working on a scale between sustenance and industrial.

It's not backward-thinking to believe that this way is better; rather, it's insane to think that abandoning regional agriculture is clever. Of course there are cultural reasons for wanting and adoring local food; your cuisine is part of your roots, even if your roots feed many trees, as they do here. Seasonality gives us reasons to celebrate what winter asparagus and spring apples cannot.

But philosophical factors aside, wouldn't you prefer to eat food that came from, say, your state, or one nearby? Or at least from within our national borders? Food you can touch, grown at farms you can visit? If our auto industry can have a renaissance, why can't our fruit-and-vegetable production?

We've seen that nothing is guaranteed: not energy, not water, not the financial system, not even the climate. Our food supply isn't guaranteed either (remember the global food shortages of 2008?), but it's more likely to provide us with security if we focus more on regional agriculture and less on trade.

NOVEMBER 1, 2011

Lawns into Gardens

The seed catalogs have arrived, and for the roughly 15 percent of Americans who appreciate the joys and rewards of growing some of their own crops, this is a more encouraging sign than Groundhog Day or even the reporting of pitchers and catchers to spring training.

Yet several times a year we hear of a situation like the one in Orlando, where the mayor claims to be striving to make his city green while his city harasses homeowners like Jason and Jennifer Helvenston for planting vegetables in their front yard, threatening to fine them $500 a day—for gardening. The battle has been raging for months, and the city's latest proposal is to allow no more than 25 percent of a homeowner's front yard to be planted in fruits and vegetables. Another example: In 2011 a Michigan woman was threatened with three months in jail for refusing to remove a vegetable garden from her front yard.

As if gardens were somehow an official eyesore, or inappropriate. (Jason Helvenston, my hero, said: "You'll take my house before you take my vegetable garden.") If you want to plant a lawn, that's fine, though it's a waste of water and energy, both petrochemical and human. Nor are lawns simply benign: many common lawn chemicals are banned in other countries, because most if not all are toxic in a variety of ways. My guess is that 100 years from now, lawns will be about as common as Hummers.

True, a lawn is a living, growing thing, a better carbon sink than concrete (though not as good as a vegetable garden or a meadow), and even more so if you leave the clippings in place, which also reduces the need for chemical fertilizer. And most people find a well-tended lawn pleasant-looking.

But when it comes to the eye of the beholder, weeds are the same thing as beauty: to a gardener, grass is a weed; a row of lettuce surrounded by dark, grassless soil a thing of beauty. To some gardeners, including me, dandelions are a crop.

The situation, then, is not black-and-white. A yard is not either unproductive and "beautiful"—as a lawn—or, as a garden, productive and "ugly." Many of us can thrill to the look of dead stalks, and even enjoy watching them rot. This is a matter of taste, not regulation.

"In a way, that's what these battles are about," says Fritz Haeg, the Los Angeles artist who initiated Edible Estates and wrote the book of the same name (subtitled "Attack on the Front Lawn"). "They're about reconsidering our basic value systems and ideas of beauty."

They're also about a relationship between us and nature. Lawns are an attempt to dominate and homogenize nature, something that hasn't worked out very well. Gardens, however, especially urban ones, make visible "the intimate relationship between people, cities, and food, constantly reminding us of the complexities and poetry of growing food and eating," says Haeg. From which, just about everyone who's thought about the subject agrees, we've all become alienated.

And small-scale suburban and urban gardening has incredible potential. Using widely available data, Roger Doiron of Kitchen Gardeners International estimates that converting 10 percent of our nation's lawns to vegetable gardens "could meet about a third of our fresh vegetable needs at current consumption rates."

Ten percent is optimistic; even 1 percent would be a terrific start, because there is a lot of lawn in this country. In fact it's our biggest crop, three times as big as corn, according to research done using a variety of data, much of it from satellites. That's around a trillion square feet—50,000 square miles—and, since an average gardener can produce something like a half-pound of food per square foot (you garden 100 square feet, you produce 50 pounds of food), without getting too geeky you can imagine that Doiron's estimates are rational.

Lawns are not exactly the enemy, but they're certainly not helping matters any. When they were used for grazing sheep—sheep are the best lawnmowers—they made some sense. But as ornamentation, only a few parts of the United States have the climate to sustain them. (Kentucky bluegrass is not even native to Kentucky, let alone Arizona.) In the remainder they're horrible water-wasters and enormous users of chemical fertilizers.

I'm not going to argue that we should be limiting the size or number of lawns, though of course plenty of municipalities already regulate the amount of water you can waste on them. In the southwest, where water is harder to come by, there has been a gradual move away from the lawn and toward the xeriscape, which simply means a more environmentally friendly ornamental yard, one that uses amounts of water appropriate to the locale. In other words, you grow cactus. And some cities, as diverse as Santa Monica, Detroit, and Portland, OR, help residents who wish to convert lawns to gardens.

Gardening may be private or a community activity; people garden together on common land, and most gardeners I know share the bounty freely. (In parts of England and France, people grow vegetables in their front yards and encourage their neighbors to take them.)

In any case there's little question that a stronger kitchen garden movement would both produce better food and put more of us in touch with where food really comes from, and how. Michelle Obama was not the first First Lady to plant a garden; Eleanor Roosevelt did it in 1943, when 20 million "victory" gardens (out of a population of only 135 million people), produced 40 percent of our fruits and vegetables. I recognize that it will take a near-apocalypse to see those kinds of numbers again, I recognize that turning lawns into gardens isn't a panacea, but I also recognize that hounding people for growing vegetables in their front yards is hardly the American way.

JANUARY 29, 2013

Celebrate the Farmer!

I recently attended a farm dinner in Maine, a long table of 60 people eating corn, chicken, salad, a spectacular herb sorbet, and other goodies. When one of the hosts arose to ask someone to describe the first course on the table—huge marrow bones from the farm's cattle—she introduced not the chef but the farmers. Similarly, at a fund-raiser on Cape Cod a week or so earlier, the talk was all about the provenance of the produce and meat rather than the cooking technique. The most popular guy was the oyster grower.

This is a fine trend. With all due respect to my chef friends (many of whom will agree with this statement), most cooking is dead-easy and pretty quick: it takes 20 minutes to roast a marrow bone, and an ambitious fifth-grader can get it right on the first try. A more complicated dish, like the seared corn with chorizo that was served a bit later, might consume an hour and require a bit of skill.

But raising and butchering the cows and pigs that produced the marrow bones and meat for the chorizo? Growing the corn? These are tasks that take weeks, if not months, of daily activity and maintenance. Like anything else, you can get good at it, but the challenges that nature and the market throw at you are never even close to being under control in the same way that a cook controls the kitchen.

What a cook doesn't control is ingredients, and that's where the debt to farmers comes in. In the last 10 or 15 years, we've seen the best New York chefs scouring the Greenmarket weekly and setting up exclusive relationships with farmers throughout the Northeast; that kind of behavior is nationwide. And even before that, Alice Waters hired people full-time to make sure the ingredients her people cooked with were the best.

The cry will ring out: Not everyone can afford fresh fruits and vegetables, especially from farm stands! And, sadly, it's true. But this is precisely why we need to support a herd of actions that will make it possible for more people to have access to real food:

We need to reduce unemployment and increase the minimum wage (including that for farm and restaurant workers). This (obviously) goes beyond the realm of food, but it's key to improving the quality of life for many if not most Americans.

We need to not cut but raise the amount of support we give to recipients of food stamps. A good example is New York City's Health Bucks program, where food stamps are worth more at farmers' markets (which don't, as a rule, sell sugar-sweetened beverages!).

We need not only to attack the nonsensical and wasteful system that pays for corn and soybeans to be grown to create junk food and ethanol, but to support local and national legislation that encourages the birth of new small-and-medium farms. We need to encourage both new and established farms to grow a variety of fruits and vegetables, to raise animals in sensible ways and, using a combination of modern and time-tested techniques, treat those animals well and use their products sensibly.

In short, we need more real farmers, not businessmen riding on half-million-dollar combines. And if you haven't seen a real farmer, go visit a one- or two-acre intensive garden; it's a mind-blowing thing, how much can be grown in a relatively small space. Then imagine thousands of 10-, 20-, and 100-acre farms planted similarly: the vegetables sold regionally, the pigs fed from scraps, the compost fertilizing the soil, the cattle at pasture, the milk making cheese . . .

The naysayers will yell, "this mode of farming will not produce enough corn and soy to feed our junk food and cheeseburger habit," and that's exactly the point. It would produce enough food so that we can all eat well. It'd produce enough food so we can slow the hysteria about our inability to feed the expected 9 billion earthlings. After all, we're not doing such a great job of feeding the current 7 billion. Why? Largely because too many resources go into producing junk food and animal products.

The Northeast, where everything but dairy farming was left for dead a decade ago, and where many dairy farmers hold on for dear life, was once its own breadbasket; sometimes it feels as if it can become that again. Local food grown by local farmers is a wonderful thing; more food grown by farmers who sell regionally brings a level of practicality to the system. Boats and trains from all over the Northeast once supplied New York City (obviously incapable of pro-ducing much in the way of truly "local" food, unless you envision re-converting Westchester, Nassau, Bergen, and Fairfield counties to farmland) with food that was picked during the day, shipped at night, and sold the next day. By com-parison, the parsley sitting in your supermarket right now is at least a week old and probably older, barring some incredible good fortune.

Real farmers, like gardeners, take pride in every tomato. And while agribusi-ness continues to try to find a way to produce a decent-tasting tomato, anyone who wants to can buy tomatoes and other fantastic produce until Thanksgiv-ing, and—in much of the country and without much effort—well into the early winter. The thrill of seasonality—not only real tomatoes but firm eggplants and cucumbers with super flavor and minimal seeds, arugula that demonstrates why it was once called rocket, peaches with loads of fuzz, and so on—reminds me why I don't often buy those things out of season.

But to get these beautiful veggies, we need real farmers who grow real food, and the will to reform a broken food system. And for that, we need not only to celebrate farmers, but also to advocate for them.

AUGUST 21, 2012

Abundance Doesn't Mean Health

The relatively new notion that around a third or more of the world's population is badly ("mal") nourished conflates hunger and diet-spawned illnesses like diabetes, both of which are preventable.

Both result from a lack of access to quality food, which in turn can result from a lack of money. No one with money starves, and the obesity-diabetes epidemic afflicts predominantly people on the low end of the income scale. With money comes good food, food that creates health and not "illth," to use John Ruskin's word. With a lack of money comes either not enough food or so-called empty calories, calories that put on pounds but do not nourish.

This is made very clear in Oxfam's "Good Enough to Eat" index, a snapshot of the state of eating in 125 countries. The index attempts to determine the best and worst countries in which to eat, by measuring levels of undernourishment and underweight in children; asking "do people have enough to eat?"; measuring costs of food versus other goods and services, to see whether food is affordable; looking at the diversity of people's diets and the availability of safe water; and monitoring diabetes and obesity levels to learn whether the diets are healthy.

The results for the United States make a fine case for American exceptionalism, though not in the way chauvinists will find pleasing.

We rank first in food affordability; food is cheap compared with other things we buy, and prices are relatively stable. We also rank highly (4th) in food "quality," which is measured by (potential) diversity of diet, though access to good water is shockingly low (tied for 41st, about a third of the way down the list).

Then the hammer falls: When it comes to healthy eating as measured by diabetes and obesity rates, we're 120th: sixth from the bottom, better off only than Saudi Arabia, Kuwait, Jordan, Fiji, and our unlucky neighbor Mexico. (Canada fares a little better; it's 18th worst.) We're also in a tie (with Belarus and other powerhouses) for 35th in "enough to eat." Really.

In fact, it's hard to imagine having a food supply as abundant as ours and doing a worse job with it. There are reasons for this:

- Much of what's grown with the potential to become "food" is actually turned into (as Michael Pollan dubbed them) edible food-like substances—in short, junk food—that produce the opposite of health. (About this there can barely be an argument any longer.) Some of what we grow is also turned into fuel for automobiles, doing no one but corn farmers any good. And much of it is fed to animals, in itself not a terrible thing, although the way we do it is damaging on many fronts.

- While we generally manage to keep the neediest quarter of our population from actually starving, we do not reach everyone who could use help; for example, only half of those Californians eligible for food stamps (officially known as the Supplemental Nutrition Assistance Program) actually get them, according to Roots of Change, a California nonprofit that focuses on food. And, of course, food stamps can be and often are used to buy junk, a pattern that causes as many problems as it alleviates.

- The budget for food education in the United States pales compared with the marketing budget for junk food, and much of that education is either unconvincing or ignored in the face of the barrage of "fun to eat" ads for the food that is worst for us. There is, as I've complained before, no concerted effort to teach people how to cook, which cannot happen without simultaneously teaching people how to shop for real food.

There are also issues of economic justice and education, and all their complications, which is why talking about food and eating inevitably leads to talking about the structure of society.

Part of the problem lies in oversight. Although we have a first lady who cares about these issues (and presumably has the support of the president), we do not have an official government policy or agency responsible for coordinating and assuring that the nation's investment in food and agriculture is for a nourishing and healthful food supply. The Department of Agriculture partly fills that role, but it also has a clear conflict of interest, since its primary goal is to support what has become a system of industrial agriculture that cares more about production and marketing supports than about what happens to soil, water, and air, or the health of consumers who buy its products. (One need look only at budgets to determine what any individual or agency cares about most.)

In the long run, what's needed is not a Farm Bill—that tangled mess that was stalled in Congress for years, and finally passed in 2014—but a national food and health policy, one that sets goals first for healthful eating and only then determines how best to produce the food that will allow us to meet those goals. It doesn't make sense to tell people to eat vegetables and then produce junk; that leads only to bad health in the face of evident abundance. What's so great about that?

JANUARY 21, 2014

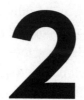

What's Wrong with
Meat?

To satisfy America's unrivaled appetite for meat and dairy, we raise and kill 10 billion animals every year. At that scale, egregious abuse (torture isn't too strong a word) is all but inevitable, while the routine use of antibiotics required to sustain such an unnatural system has become a public health menace. Despite the best (and sometimes preposterous) efforts of industrial meat producers to hide inhumane and dangerous practices from consumers, the horrors of factory farming have been well documented.

Vastly improving this system requires action on multiple fronts: meat distributors and producers mandating better living conditions for animals; the F.D.A. cracking down on antibiotics; increased support (both governmental and personal) for farms that value animal welfare as much or more than the bottom line. Progress is being made, but slowly.

Of course, the best way to protect animals is to consume fewer of them. It's that simple, and while meaningfully curbing the country's demand for meat could take decades, you can start doing your part at the dinner table tonight. In this chapter, a look at both the problems and the potential solutions.

Rethinking the Meat Guzzler

A sea change in the consumption of a resource that Americans take for granted may be in store—something cheap, plentiful, widely enjoyed, and a part of daily life. And it isn't oil.

It's meat.

The two commodities share a great deal: Like oil, meat is subsidized by the federal government. Like oil, meat is subject to accelerating demand as nations become wealthier, and this, in turn, sends prices higher. Finally—like oil—meat is something people are encouraged to consume less of, as the toll exacted by industrial production increases, and becomes increasingly visible.

Global demand for meat has multiplied in recent years, encouraged by growing affluence and nourished by the proliferation of huge, confined animal feeding operations. These assembly-line meat factories consume enormous amounts of energy, pollute water supplies, generate significant greenhouse gases, and require ever-increasing amounts of corn, soy, and other grains, a dependency that has led to the destruction of vast swaths of the world's tropical rain forests.

The president of Brazil has announced emergency measures to halt the burning and cutting of the country's rain forests for crop and grazing land. In the last five months alone, the government says, 1,250 square miles were lost.

The world's total meat supply was 71 million tons in 1961. In 2007, it was estimated to be 284 million tons. Per capita consumption has more than doubled over that period. (In the developing world, it rose twice as fast, doubling in the last 20 years.) World meat consumption is expected to double again by 2050, which one expert, Henning Steinfeld of the United Nations, says is resulting in a "relentless growth in livestock production."

Americans eat about the same amount of meat as we have for some time, about eight ounces a day, roughly twice the global average. At about 5 percent of the world's population, we "process" (that is, grow and kill) nearly 10 billion animals a year, more than 15 percent of the world's total.

Growing meat (it's hard to use the word "raising" when applied to animals in factory farms) uses so many resources that it's a challenge to enumerate them all. But consider: an estimated 30 percent of the earth's ice-free land is directly or indirectly involved in livestock production, according to the United Nations Food and Agriculture Organization, which also estimates that livestock production generates nearly a fifth of the world's greenhouse gases—more than transportation.

To put the energy-using demand of meat production into easy-to-understand terms, Gidon Eshel, a geophysicist at the Bard Center, and Pamela A. Martin, an assistant professor of geophysics at the University of Chicago, calculated that if Americans were to reduce meat consumption by just 20 percent it would be as if we all switched from a standard sedan—a Camry, say—to the ultra-efficient Prius. Similarly, a study last year by the National Institute of Livestock and Grassland Science in Japan estimated that 2.2 pounds of beef is responsible for the equivalent amount of carbon dioxide emitted by the average European car every 155 miles, and burns enough energy to light a 100-watt bulb for nearly 20 days.

Grain, meat, and even energy are roped together in a way that could have dire results. More meat means a corresponding increase in demand for feed, especially corn and soy, which some experts say will contribute to higher prices.

This will be inconvenient for citizens of wealthier nations, but it could have tragic consequences for those of poorer ones, especially if higher prices for feed divert production away from food crops. The demand for ethanol is already pushing up prices, and explains, in part, the 40 percent rise last year in the food price index calculated by the United Nations Food and Agriculture Organization.

Though some 800 million people on the planet now suffer from hunger or malnutrition, the majority of corn and soy grown in the world feeds cattle, pigs, and chickens. This despite the inherent inefficiencies: about two to five times more grain is required to produce the same amount of calories through livestock as through direct grain consumption, according to Rosamond Naylor, an associate professor of economics at Stanford University. It is as much as 10 times more in the case of grain-fed beef in the United States.

The environmental impact of growing so much grain for animal feed is profound. Agriculture in the United States—much of which now serves the demand for meat—contributes to nearly three-quarters of all water-quality problems in the nation's rivers and streams, according to the Environmental Protection Agency.

Because the stomachs of cattle are meant to digest grass, not grain, cattle raised industrially thrive only in the sense that they gain weight quickly. This diet made it possible to remove cattle from their natural environment and encourage the efficiency of mass confinement and slaughter. But it causes enough health problems that administration of antibiotics is routine, so much so that it can result in antibiotic-resistant bacteria that threaten the usefulness of medicines that treat people.

Those grain-fed animals, in turn, are contributing to health problems among the world's wealthier citizens—heart disease, some types of cancer, diabetes. The argument that meat provides useful protein makes sense, if the quantities are small. But the "you gotta eat meat" claim collapses at American levels. Even if the amount of meat we eat weren't harmful, it's way more than enough.

Americans are downing close to 200 pounds of meat, poultry, and fish per capita per year (dairy and eggs are separate, and hardly insignificant), an increase of 50 pounds per person from 50 years ago. We each consume something like 110 grams of protein a day, about twice the federal government's recommended allowance; of that, about 75 grams come from animal protein. (The recommended level is itself considered by many dietary experts to be higher than it needs to be.) It's likely that most of us would do just fine on around 30 grams of protein a day, virtually all of it from plant sources.

What can be done? There's no simple answer. Better waste management, for one. Eliminating subsidies would also help; the United Nations estimates that they account for 31 percent of global farm income. Improved farming practices would help, too. Mark W. Rosegrant, director of environment and production technology at the nonprofit International Food Policy Research Institute, says, "There should be investment in livestock breeding and management, to reduce the footprint needed to produce any given level of meat."

Then there's technology. Israel and Korea are among the countries experimenting with using animal waste to generate electricity. Some of the biggest hog operations in the United States are working, with some success, to turn manure into fuel.

Longer term, it no longer seems lunacy to believe in the possibility of "meat without feet"—meat produced in vitro, by growing animal cells in a super-rich nutrient environment before being further manipulated into burgers and steaks.

Another suggestion is a return to grazing beef, a very real alternative as long as you accept the psychologically difficult and politically unpopular notion of eating less of it. That's because grazing could never produce as many cattle as feedlots do. Still, said Michael Pollan, author of *In Defense of Food*, "In places where you can't grow grain, fattening cows on grass is always going to make more sense."

But pigs and chickens, which convert grain to meat far more efficiently than beef, are increasingly the meats of choice for producers, accounting for 70 percent of total meat production, with industrialized systems producing half the pork and three-quarters of the chicken.

Once, these animals were raised locally (even many New Yorkers remember the pigs of Secaucus), reducing transportation costs and allowing their manure to be spread on nearby fields. Now hog production facilities that resemble prisons more than farms are hundreds of miles from major population centers, and their manure "lagoons" pollute streams and groundwater. (In Iowa alone, hog factories and farms produce more than 50 million tons of excrement annually.)

These problems originated here, but are no longer limited to the United States. While the domestic demand for meat has leveled off, the industrial production of livestock is growing more than twice as fast as land-based methods, according to the United Nations.

Perhaps the best hope for change lies in consumers' becoming aware of the true costs of industrial meat production. "When you look at environmental problems in the U.S.," says Professor Eshel, "nearly all of them have their source in food production and in particular meat production. And factory farming is 'optimal' only as long as degrading waterways is free. If dumping this stuff becomes costly—even if it simply carries a non-zero price tag—the entire structure of food production will change dramatically."

Animal welfare may not yet be a major concern, but as the horrors of raising meat in confinement become known, more animal lovers may start to react. And would the world not be a better place were some of the grain we use to grow meat directed instead to feed our fellow human beings?

Real prices of beef, pork, and poultry have held steady, perhaps even decreased, for 40 years or more (in part because of grain subsidies), though we're beginning to see them increase now. But many experts, including Tyler Cowen, a professor of economics at George Mason University, say they don't believe meat prices will rise high enough to affect demand in the United States.

"I just don't think we can count on market prices to reduce our meat consumption," he said. "There may be a temporary spike in food prices, but it will almost certainly be reversed and then some. But if all the burden is put on eaters, that's not a tragic state of affairs."

If price spikes don't change eating habits, perhaps the combination of deforestation, pollution, climate change, starvation, heart disease, and animal cruelty will gradually encourage the simple daily act of eating more plants and fewer animals.

Mr. Rosegrant of the Food Policy Research Institute says he foresees "a stronger public relations campaign in the reduction of meat consumption—one like that around cigarettes—emphasizing personal health, compassion for animals, and doing good for the poor and the planet."

It wouldn't surprise Professor Eshel if all of this had a real impact. "The good of people's bodies and the good of the planet are more or less perfectly aligned," he said.

The United Nations' Food and Agriculture Organization, in its detailed 2006 study of the impact of meat consumption on the planet, "Livestock's Long Shadow," made a similar point: "There are reasons for optimism that the conflicting demands for animal products and environmental services can be reconciled. Both demands are exerted by the same group of people . . . the relatively affluent, middle- to high-income class, which is no longer confined to industrialized countries. . . . This group of consumers is probably ready to use its growing voice to exert pressure for change and may be willing to absorb the inevitable price increases."

In fact, Americans are already buying more environmentally friendly products, choosing more sustainably produced meat, eggs, and dairy. The number of farmers' markets has more than doubled in the last 10 years or so, and it has escaped no one's notice that the organic food market is growing fast. These all represent products that are more expensive but of higher quality.

If those trends continue, meat may become a treat rather than a routine. It won't be uncommon, but just as surely as the S.U.V. will yield to the hybrid, the half-pound-a-day meat era will end.

We're Eating Less Meat. Why?

Americans eat more meat than any other population in the world; about one-sixth of the total, though we're less than one-twentieth of the population.

But that's changing.

Until recently, almost everyone considered their dinner plate naked without a big old hunk of meat on it. (You remember "Beef: It's What's for Dinner," of course. How could you forget?) And we could afford it: our production methods and the denial of their true costs have kept meat cheap beyond all credibility. (American hamburger is arguably the cheapest convenience food there is.) This, in part, is why we spend a smaller percentage of our money on food than any other country, and much of that goes toward the roughly half-pound of meat each of us eats, on average, every day.

But that's changing, and considering the fairly steady climb in meat consumption over the last half-century, you might say the numbers are plummeting. The Department of Agriculture projects that our meat and poultry consumption will fall again this year, to about 12.2 percent less in 2012 than it was in 2007. Beef consumption has been in decline for about 20 years; the drop in chicken is even more dramatic, over the last five years or so; pork also has been steadily slipping for about five years.

The report treats consumers as victims of government bias against the meat industry. We're eating less meat because we want to eat less meat.

Holy cow. What's up?

It's easy enough to round up the usual suspects, which is what a story in the *Daily* did last month. It blames the decline on growing exports, which make less meat available for Americans to buy. It blames it on ethanol, which has caused feed costs to rise, production to drop, and prices to go up so producers can cover their increasing costs. It blames drought. It doesn't blame recession, which is surprising, because that's a factor also.

All of which makes some sense. The report then goes on to blame the federal government for "wag[ing] war on meat protein consumption" over the last 30-40 years.

Is this like the war on drugs? The war in Afghanistan? The war against cancer? Because what I see here is:

- a history of subsidies for the corn and soy that's fed to livestock

- a nearly free pass on environmental degradation and animal abuse

- an unwillingness to meaningfully limit the use of antibiotics in animal feed

- a failure to curb the stifling power that corporate meatpackers wield over smaller ranchers

- and what amounts to a refusal—despite the advice of real, disinterested experts, true scientists in fact—to unequivocally advise consumers that they should be eating less meat

Or is the occasional environmental protection regulation and whisper that unlimited meat at every meal might not be ideal the equivalent of war? Is the U.S.D.A. buying $40 million worth of chicken products to reduce the surplus and raise retail prices the equivalent of war?

No. It's not the non-existent federal War on Meat that's making a difference. And even if availability is down, it's not as if we're going to the supermarket and finding empty meat cases and deli counters filled with coleslaw. The flaw in the report is that it treats American consumers as passive actors who are victims of diminishing supplies, rising costs, and government bias against the meat industry. Nowhere does it mention that we're eating less meat because we want to eat less meat.

Yet conscious decisions are being made by consumers. Even buying less meat because prices are high and times are tough is a choice; other "sacrifices" could be made. We could cut back on junk food, or shirts, or iPhones, which have a very high meat-equivalent, to coin a term. Yet even though excess supply kept chicken prices lower than the year before, demand dropped.

Some are choosing to eat less meat for all the right reasons. The Values Institute at DGWB Advertising and Communications just named the rise of "flexitarianism"—an eating style that reduces the amount of meat without "going vegetarian"—as one of its top five consumer health trends for 2012. In an Allrecipes.com survey of 1,400 members, more than one-third of home cooks said they ate less meat in 2011 than in 2010. Back in June, a survey found that 50 percent of American adults said they were aware of the Meatless Monday campaign, with 27 percent of those aware reporting that they were actively reducing their meat consumption.

I can add, anecdotally, that when I ask audiences I speak to, "How many of you are eating less meat than you were 10 years ago?" at least two-thirds raise their hands. A self-selecting group to be sure, but nevertheless one that exists.

In fact, let's ask this: is anyone in this country eating more meat than they used to?

We still eat way more meat than is good for us or the environment, not to mention the animals. But a 12 percent reduction in just five years is significant, and if that decline were to continue for the next five years—well, that's something few would have imagined five years ago. It's something only the industry could get upset about. The rest of us should celebrate. Rice and beans, anyone?

JANUARY 10, 2012

Banned from the Barn

Iowa's ag-gag law failed to pass before summer recess last week: a good thing. The ridiculous proposition, which died along with similar ones in Minnesota, Florida, and New York, would have made it illegal to videotape or photograph in the agricultural facilities that house almost all of our chickens and pigs.

Sadly, a lack of idiocy is not the same thing as a presence of wisdom, and the demise of ag-gag won't give us a clearer view of food production. We need more visibility, not less. But when I visited Iowa in May, I appealed to producers of eggs, chickens, pork, and even cooking oil to let me visit their facilities. In general, I was ignored, politely refused, or told something like "it's a bad week." (I made standing offers to return at any time; no one has taken me up on that.)

When a journalist can't see how the food we eat is produced, you don't need ag-gag laws. The system's already gagged.

The videographers that have made it into closed barns have revealed that eggs are laid and chickens are born and raised in closed barns containing (literally) hundreds of thousands of birds; an outsider wouldn't even know what those barns were. Pigs are housed cheek-to-jowl, by the many thousands, in what are called concentrated animal feeding operations, where feeding, watering, and monitoring are largely mechanized. Pregnant sows are confined in small concrete cells. Iowa is industrial agriculture's ground zero. But when it comes to producing animals, zero is pretty much what you're going to see.

One medium-size pig-raising operation did offer me a tour, and we drove to a site where they ran four barns, each of which normally housed around 1,200 pigs. But the one we explored held only 200 pigs and reeked of deodorant. The animals had plenty of room, and they were calm and clean, as were the floors.

Not at all what I expected. Except I'd been expected, and a cleanup must have preceded me by, I'd guess, no more than two hours. (Either that or these were magic, non-defecating pigs.)

"Where are the other thousand pigs?" I asked.

"We've shipped a whole bunch recently."

"How about the other three barns? Are they full?"

"Nope. We don't have many pigs here right now."

Some tour. But I'd seen other pig barns during the course of the week because whenever I saw one that appeared unattended (it's easy enough to tell; there's no car), I checked it out as best I could. On some roads, there are almost as many pig barns as farmhouses, which may not be a coincidence: If you were an older farmer and your neighbor put 1,200 pigs in a barn, you'd probably move to Florida, too. The smell can be overwhelming.

Most have a small enclosure by the road, usually with a Dumpster. That's where dead pigs are tossed until the next garbage collection. (Yes, I saw this, several times.) Many of the barns are open on the sides so you can see how crowded the pigs are. (Videos of gestation barns—virtually impossible for an outsider to see—show that the sows can't even turn around.) The pigs were visibly upset when I approached the outside of the barn.

That was the best I could do, and it wasn't much. I could've been arrested for trespassing; extreme versions of ag-gag would make it illegal for me to write about it, or at least publish pictures.

Which would bring us a step closer to China, whose Health Ministry is trying to clamp down on news media outlets that "mislead" the public about food safety issues. (It's worth noting, on the other hand, that the Chinese Supreme Court has called for the death penalty in cases of fatal food poisoning.) "Mislead" apparently means reporting about pork tainted with the banned drug clenbuterol, which sent a couple hundred wedding guests to the hospital; watermelons exploding from the overuse of chemicals; pork disguised as beef, or glowing blue; and—my favorite—cooking oil dredged from sewers.

Our watermelons don't explode and, for now, I can write about it. Yet when a heroic videographer breaks a horror story about animal cruelty, as happens every month or so, the industry writes off the offense as an isolated incident, and the perpetrators—usually the workers, who are "just following orders"—

are fired or given wrist slaps. Business continues as usual, and it will until the public better understands industrial animal-rearing techniques.

"When I grew up here," said an Iowan I spent some time with, "people were proud of their animals. They'd have signs with their breeds, or their names, and they'd offer to show you around." That's no longer the case with most animal operations in Iowa.

JULY 6, 2011

Some Animals Are More Equal Than Others

I t's time to take a look at the line between "pet" and "animal." When the ASPCA sends an agent to the home of a Brooklyn family to arrest one of its members for allegedly killing a hamster, something is wrong.

That "something" is this: we protect "companion animals" like hamsters while largely ignoring what amounts to the torture of chickens and cows and pigs. In short, if I keep a pig as a pet, I can't kick it. If I keep a pig I intend to sell for food, I can pretty much torture it. State laws known as "Common Farming Exemptions" allow industry—rather than lawmakers—to make any practice legal as long as it's common. "In other words," as Jonathan Safran Foer, the author of *Eating Animals*, wrote me via e-mail, "the industry has the power to define cruelty. It's every bit as crazy as giving burglars the power to define trespassing."

Meanwhile, there are pet police. So when 19-year-old Monique Smith slammed her sibling's hamster on the floor and killed it, as she may have done in a fit of rage last week, an ASPCA agent—there are 18 of them, busily responding to animal cruelty calls in the five boroughs and occasionally beyond—arrested her. (The charges were later dropped, though Ms. Smith spent a night in jail at Rikers Island.)

In light of the way most animals are treated in this country, I'm pretty sure that ASPCA agents don't need to spend their time in Brooklyn defending rodents.

In fact, there's no rationality to be found here. Just a few blocks from Ms. Smith's home, along the M subway line, the city routinely is poisoning rodents as quickly and futilely as it possibly can, though rats can be pets also. But that's hardly the point. This is: we "process" (that means kill) nearly 10 billion animals annually in this country, approximately one-sixth of the world's total.

Many if not most of these animals are raised (or not, since probably a couple of hundred million are killed at birth) industrially, in conditions that the philosopher Peter Singer and others have compared to concentration camps. Might we more usefully police those who keep egg-laying hens in cages so small the birds can't open their wings, for example, than anger-management-challenged young people accused of hamstercide?

Yet Ms. Smith was charged as a felon, because in New York (and there are similar laws in other states) if you kick a dog or cat or hamster or, I suppose, a guppy, enough to "cause extreme physical pain" or do so "in an especially depraved or sadistic manner" you may be guilty of aggravated cruelty to animals, as long as you do this "with no justifiable purpose."

But thanks to Common Farming Exemptions, as long as I "raise" animals for food and it's done by my fellow "farmers" (in this case, manufacturers might be a better word), I can put around 200 million male chicks a year through grinders, castrate—mostly without anesthetic—65 million calves and piglets a year, breed sick animals (don't forget: more than half a billion eggs were recalled last summer, from just two Iowa farms) who in turn breed antibiotic-resistant bacteria, allow those sick animals to die without individual veterinary care, imprison animals in cages so small they cannot turn around, skin live animals, or kill animals en masse to stem disease outbreaks.

All of this is legal, because we will eat them.

We have "justifiable purposes": pleasure (or, at this point, habit, because eating is hardly a pleasure if you do it in your car, or in 10 minutes), convenience—there are few things more filling per dollar than a cheeseburger—and of course corporate profits. We should be treating animals better and raising fewer of them; this would naturally reduce our consumption. All in all, a better situation for us, the animals, the world.

Arguing for the freedom to eat as much meat as you want is equivalent to arguing for treating farm animals as if they could not feel pain. Yet no one would defend Ms. Smith's cruel action because it was a pet and therefore not born to be put through living hell.

Is it really that bad? After all, a new video from Smithfield, the world's largest pork producer, makes industrial pig-raising seem like a little bit of heaven. But undercover videos from the Humane Society of the United States tell quite a different story, and a repulsive one. It also explains why we saw laws proposed by friends of agribusiness in both Iowa and Florida in recent weeks that would ban making such videos: the truth hurts, especially if you support the status quo.

Our fantasy is that until the industrial era domesticated animals were treated decently. Maybe that's true, and maybe it isn't; but certainly they weren't turned out by the tens of thousands as if they were widgets.

We're finally seeing some laws that take the first steps toward generally ameliorating cruelty to farm animals, and it's safe to say that most of today's small farmers and even some larger ones raise animals humanely. These few, at least, are treated with as much respect as the law believes we should treat a hamster.

For the majority of non-pets, though, it's tough luck.

MARCH 15, 2011

On Becoming
China's Farm Team

Look at the $4.7 billion purchase of the pork producer Smithfield Foods by Shuanghui International Holdings Ltd.—the Chinese firm that counts Goldman Sachs among its backers—from the standpoint of the Chinese. As this century's economic titan, they had to "take a position" in United States pork. China's population of nearly 1.4 billion is not only growing rapidly but growing wealthier rapidly, and flattering us by emulating our consumption patterns (for better or worse) while having trouble replicating some of our production systems.

China has notorious problems with food safety; urban Chinese consumers distrust the quality and safety of their own food system, and express clear preference for imported food when it is available. What to do when you are the largest pork supplier in China, you have production and quality problems, must meet the ravenous demand for more meat from hundreds of millions of paying consumers, and the international supply is abundant? You buy producer and processor, together with that firm's vaunted supply chain, quality controls, brand value, and consumer appeal.

Sadly, there may be only one potential upside to this deal for most Americans, and that one is ironic. We might see a marginal improvement in the quality of industrially produced pork by ridding it of ractopamine, a lean-meat growth stimulant whose effects on humans are sufficiently questionable that its use for meat production is illegal in the European Union, Russia, and China. Smithfield says that as of June, 50 percent of its pork is ractopamine-free, the better to please its new masters.

But can Americans buy Smithfield pork without ractopamine? Maybe, maybe not. At the moment, there's no way to know.

The other upsides are for the Chinese, and of course, Smithfield share-holders, though Smithfield executives would have you believe otherwise. Larry Pope, Smithfield's C.E.O., who is no doubt glowing about what turned out to be a $34-per-share premium, told the Senate committee on Agriculture, Nutrition, and Forestry that the purchase—the biggest ever of a United States company by a Chinese one—"provides enormous benefits . . . for American manufacturing and agriculture," and claims it will result in more production, jobs, and exports.

"It'll be the same old Smithfield, only better," Mr. Pope said.

The Chinese produce and consume half the world's pigs. They have a pork strategic reserve not unlike our petroleum reserve. Really. They'll buy more pork from us when they can and need to, but not simply because a Chinese company owns the factory. (Would you, for example, be more likely to buy a Kia if Goldman Sachs bought the Korean carmaker? For that matter, can you be certain that they haven't?) If they did, and pork became scarcer, prices would climb; producers might consider that a good thing but consumers would not. Almost anything that reduces consumption of industrially produced meat is a plus, but reducing its production is equally important, and there's the rub, or one of them.

The benefits for Shuanghui are crystal clear: As is the case with 90 percent of the pork produced in the United States, almost all of Smithfield's "farms" use now standard techniques, including large (average: 2,000 pigs) concentrated animal feeding operations, or CAFOs, in which pigs are confined, fed with legal but problematic drugs, and use enormous amounts of feed, water, and energy while generating giant lagoons of manure. (That Smithfield has made some progress in manure disposal and even confinement are minor if not insignificant factors when the entire production model is assessed.)

Smithfield has also bred what might be the world's leanest and therefore most profitable pork, using genetic research paid for in part with tax dollars through public support of research at land-grant universities. Technologically speaking, the almost inconceivably huge Chinese pork industry is primitive. This is an instantaneous technology transfer that doesn't involve spying but cash.

Given what they just outsourced, why would the Chinese not want to buy the whole shebang? According to Kai Olson-Sawyer, a research and policy analyst at the Grace Communications Foundation, "The CAFO system has major impacts on environmental and human health, rural communities, and animal welfare. And basically, taxpayers pay for it all: we subsidize the production of cheap grain used as feed, and are ultimately stuck bearing the environmental, public health, and socioeconomic costs of industrial livestock production."

The fact is that China is going to be a net importer of food more or less forever: it's got a fifth of the world's population (and eats a fifth of the world's food), but only 9 percent of its agricultural land and scarce water resources. (The average pig takes nearly 600 gallons of water to produce a pound of meat.)

So even more than a technology grab, the Smithfield deal is a land and water grab. We still have the world's most enviable combination of arable land, rainfall, and temperate weather, and there's no practical technological substitute for any of these. It's the consumption of these resources, along with the manure deposits, that make the Smithfield deal, to paraphrase Warren Buffett, a form of colonization by purchase rather than conquest. In short, the deal, as he wrote in *Fortune*, is "really about owning access to America's safe farmland and clean water supplies."

Put aside for a moment the arguments of those who see a better way to eat and produce food more sustainably. And put aside that most Americans remain ignorant of how food is produced and the effect that production has on land, water, energy, and even climate. Just say this: all agriculture has impact, which means it uses resources and leaves behind waste. We implicitly accept some of that impact because we want, for example, the pork.

The Smithfield-Shuanghui deal guarantees China the pork while offloading the downsides (the "externalities") of pork production onto The Land of the Free. It guarantees us cropland devoted to chemical-dependent monoculture; continued overuse of water and other resources, none of which we can afford to squander; and great big stinking piles of manure. In sum, it transfers the environmental damage of large-scale pork production from China to the United States without even guaranteeing us pork with as few chemicals as that shipped to China.

Welcome to China's farm team.

NOVEMBER 5, 2013

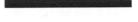

Should You Eat Chicken?

As one salmonella outbreak follows another, I'm frequently asked "Should I stop eating chicken?"

It's a good question. In recent weeks, salmonella on chicken has officially sickened more than 300 people (the Centers for Disease Control says there are 25 illnesses for every one reported, so maybe 7,500) and hospitalized more than 40 percent of them, in part because antibiotics aren't working. Industry's reaction has been predictably disappointing: the chicken from the processors in question—Foster Farms—is still being shipped into the market. Regulators' responses have been limited: the same chicken in question is still being sold.

Until the Food Safety and Inspection Service (F.S.I.S.) of the Department of Agriculture (U.S.D.A.) can get its act together and start assuring us that chicken is safe, I'd be wary.

This is not a shutdown issue, but a "We care more about industry than we do about consumers" issue. Think that's an exaggeration? Read this mission statement: "The Food Safety and Inspection Service is the public health agency in the U.S. Department of Agriculture responsible for ensuring that the nation's commercial supply of meat, poultry, and egg products is safe, wholesome, and correctly labeled and packaged." What part of "safe" am I misreading?

We should all steer clear at least of Foster Farms chicken, or any of the other brands produced in that company's California plants, although they're not all labeled as such. Costco, for example, pulled nearly 9,000 rotisserie chickens from a store south of San Francisco after finding contamination—this is after cooking, mind you—with a strain of salmonella Heidelberg, which is virulent, nasty, and resistant to some commonly used antibiotics.

In sum: 1. There's salmonella on chicken (some of which, by the way, is labeled "organic"). 2. It's making many people sick, and some antibiotics aren't working. 3. Production continues in the plants linked to the outbreak. 4. Despite warnings by many federal agencies (including itself!), the U.S.D.A. has done nothing to get these chickens out of the marketplace. 5. Even Costco can't seem to make these chickens safe to eat.

For decades, we've been told how to handle chicken. But I can tell you that despite my best efforts to keep raw chicken and its drippings quarantined, I'm not confident that these efforts suffice. What if chicken blood gets on my lettuce in a shopping bag? What if someone else's chicken contaminates my apples on a supermarket conveyor belt? What if my wife or a guest grabs a cutting board or a knife before it's been washed? These are not paranoid questions.

What if—as happened to a Florida client of Bill Marler's, the Seattle-based food safety attorney—I go to a barbecue, and I eat a piece of chicken, and I get sick? And I don't respond to antibiotics? And I wind up in the hospital with sepsis (blood poisoning) and stop breathing, and maybe have a long-term brain injury because of lack of oxygen? "All for going to a neighbor's barbecue," says Marler.

Who's at fault here? The victim, for eating chicken cooked by a neighbor? The neighbor, for not being trained in public safety? Or the producer, who won't slow down processing to guarantee safety? Or the regulator, who is "responsible for ensuring" safety?

We have to assume Costco has a pretty rigorous food safety program. And safe chicken, as we've been told ad infinitum, is chicken that's cooked to 165 degrees Fahrenheit; at that point all the salmonella on it should be dead.

Well, guess what? Costco cooks its chicken to 180 degrees Fahrenheit, a margin of error that the company believes renders the chicken safe. But that didn't work here. Which means, as far as I can tell, one of four things: the chicken wasn't cooked to 180 degrees Fahrenheit; or there was some cross-contamination; or there was so much salmonella on the birds that even "proper" cooking couldn't kill it all (this can happen; 165 degrees Fahrenheit isn't a magic number); or . . . maybe there's now a strain of salmonella that isn't killed at 165 degrees Fahrenheit.

I asked Congresswoman Louise Slaughter, Democrat of New York, who has a degree in microbiology, whether that last was possible. Her answer was immediate and unequivocal: "Of course it is." Daniel Englejohn, deputy assistant administrator at F.S.I.S., said that there is "no evidence that these strains are more resistant to heat than others." When I asked if the agency might choose to err on the side of caution, he said, "We did take an action to alert the public to safely handle and prepare their products." Wow.

To its credit, Costco pulled the rotisserie chicken from its shelves, as did a couple of other retailers. (To its debit, Costco left raw Foster Farms chicken on the shelves, once again transferring the burden of safety to the consumer, even though the store must have known that it couldn't guarantee that cooking the chicken would render it safe.) Foster Farms has not recalled a single piece of chicken, although it's arguable that this same contamination has been going on for months. And F.S.I.S. officially has no power to do so.

The agency could, however, remove its inspectors from the three suspect plants, which would close them, and last week it threatened to do just that. Three days later, Foster Farms "submitted and implemented immediate substantive changes to their slaughter and processing to allow for continued operations." What's that mean? "We cannot tell you what their interventions are, because that's a proprietary issue," said Englejohn, adding that the interventions comprise "additional sanitary measures that reduce contamination." Well, we hope so.

Meanwhile, commerce continues and the chicken is out there. Will it be taken off the market after 800 people get sick? Or 1,200? Or when someone dies? Or, as F.S.I.S. would prefer, will this just die down until the next time?

We should not have to handle chicken as if it were a loaded gun, nor should we be blamed when contaminated chicken makes us sick.

U.S.D.A. does not stand alone. The Food and Drug Administration (F.D.A.), knowing that manufacturers grow animals under conditions virtually guaranteed to breed disease, allows them to attempt to ward off disease by feeding them antibiotics from birth until death. (This despite the stated intention of the agency to change that, and a court order requiring it to.) This rampant drug use has led to new strains of bacteria that are resistant to many antibiotics. And the situation is getting worse.

Believe it or not, the presence of salmonella on chicken is both common and acceptable. (About a quarter of all chicken parts are contaminated, a fact of which F.S.I.S. is fully aware and which it is evaluating.) From the Centers for Disease Control: "It is not unusual for raw poultry from any producer to have salmonella bacteria. C.D.C. and U.S.D.A.-F.S.I.S. recommend consumers follow food safety tips to prevent salmonella infection from raw poultry produced by Foster Farms or any other brand."

Right. But if salmonella was ever easily killed by careful handling and cooking, perhaps that is no longer the case; perhaps it's more virulent and heartier, and it certainly now defies some antibiotics.

The real solution lies not only in washing your hands but in improving production methods. As Congresswoman Rosa DeLauro, Democrat of Connecticut, who, like Slaughter, is one of our best (and only) Congressional food safety advocates, said to me, "We need to reform this system."

And the reforms are pretty straightforward. If the F.D.A. and U.S.D.A. want to stand with citizens rather than industry when it comes to meat safety, there are two necessary steps.

1. The F.D.A. must disallow the use of prophylactic antibiotics in animal production. It's almost as simple as that.

2. The U.S.D.A. must consider salmonella that's been linked to illness an "adulterant" (as it does strains of E. coli), which would mean that its very presence on foods would be sufficient to take them off the market. Again, it's almost as simple as that. (Sweden produces chicken with zero levels of salmonella. Are they that much smarter than us?)

This assumes our agencies are willing to put our interests before industry's. If they're not, I guess the question "Whose side are you on?" has been answered. Meanwhile . . . should you eat chicken? That's your call.

OCTOBER 15, 2013

A Chicken Without Guilt

It is pretty well established that animals are capable of suffering; we've come a long way since Descartes famously compared them to nonfeeling machines put on earth to serve man. (Rousseau later countered this, saying that animals shared "some measure" of human nature and should partake of "natural right.") No matter where you stand on this spectrum, you probably agree that it's a noble goal to reduce the level of the suffering of animals raised for meat in industrial conditions.

There are four ways to move toward fixing this. One, we can improve the animals' living conditions; two (this is distasteful but would shock no one), we might see producers reduce or even eliminate animals' consciousness, say, by removing the cerebral cortex, in effect converting them to a kind of vegetable (see Margaret Atwood's horrifying description in her prescient *Oryx and Crake*); three, we can consume fewer industrially raised animals, concentrating on those raised more humanely.

Or four, we can reduce consumption, period. That is perhaps difficult when people eat an average of a half-pound of meat daily. But as better fake plant-based "meat" products are created, that option becomes more palatable. My personal approval of fake meat, for what it's worth, has been long in coming. I like traditional meat substitutes, like tofu, bean burgers, vegetable cutlets, and so on, but have been mostly repelled by unconvincing nuggets and hot dogs, which lack bite, chew, juiciness, and flavor. I'm also annoyed by the cost: why pay more for fake meat than real meat, especially since the production process is faster, easier, and involves no butchering? And, I have felt, if you want to eat less meat, why not just eat more of other real things?

With these thoughts in mind I visited a place in The Hague called The Vegetarian Butcher, where the "butcher" said to me, "We slaughter soy"—ha-ha. The plant-based products were actually pretty good—the chicken would have fooled me if I hadn't known what it was—and I began to consider that it might be better to eat fake meat that harms no animals and causes less environmental damage than meat raised industrially.

(When I say fake meat, I don't mean the much publicized laboratory simulacrum from Maastricht University that combines pig cells and horse fetal serum, a mixture that's then "fed" sugar, fat, amino acids, and so on, to produce translucent strips. We'll tackle that when and if it becomes marketable.)

Really: Would I rather eat cruelly raised, polluting, unhealthful chicken, or a plant product that's nutritionally similar or superior, good enough to fool me, and requires no antibiotics, cutting off of heads, or other nasty things? Isn't it preferable, at least some of the time, to eat plant products mixed with water that have been put through a thingamajiggy that spews out meatlike stuff, instead of eating those same plant products put into a chicken that does its biomechanical thing for the six weeks of its miserable existence, only to have its throat cut in the service of yielding barely distinguishable meat?

Why, in other words, use the poor chicken as a machine to produce meat when you can use a machine to produce "meat" that seems like chicken?

I love good chicken, but most of the chicken we eat doesn't qualify, and the question becomes more compelling as meat imitators gain sophistication. The vegetarian meat I ate in The Hague isn't widely distributed, but Quorn, a mushroom-based product, can be pretty appealing in some instances, Gardein has made some advances in soy-based products, and at least one new product is a better-than-adequate substitute for chicken in things like wraps, salads, and sauces. I know this because Ethan Brown, an owner of Savage, came to my house and fooled me badly in a blind tasting. (A pan-European "Like Meat" project appears to be making progress on a similar product, and others are in the works.)

On its own, Brown's "chicken"—produced to mimic boneless, skinless breast—looks like a decent imitation, and the way it shreds is amazing. It doesn't taste much like chicken, but since most white meat chicken doesn't taste like much anyway, that's hardly a problem; both are about texture, chew, and the ingredients you put on them or combine with them. When you take Brown's product, cut it up, and combine it with, say, chopped tomato and lettuce and mayonnaise with some seasoning in it, and wrap it in a burrito, you won't know the difference between that and chicken. I didn't, at least, and this is the kind of thing I do for a living. Brown does not see his product as a trendy meat replacement for vegans but one with more widespread use. (His production is at an early stage, but Whole Foods is planning to start using his products in prepared food soon. Retail sales of his "chicken," which does not yet have a trademarked name, are expected to begin this summer.)

Perhaps it will replace some of the chicken in a McNugget, or become a meat substitute at Chick-fil-A or Chipotle. (Department of Agriculture regulations already permit up to 30 percent soy products in school lunch meats.)

We're ready for this. According to a Harris poll commissioned by the Vegetarian Resource Group, a third of Americans now eat meatless meals "a significant amount of the time," and that doesn't include vegetarians, who make up at least 3 percent of the population. These numbers would grow faster, advocates of meatlike plant foods believe, if fake meat fooled us more often.

"When you 'veganize' food convincingly," says Kathy Freston, author of *Veganist: Lose Weight, Get Healthy, Change the World*, "people can enjoy a healthier, better version of their traditional favorites. And if you know that food won't hurt your body or the environment and it didn't cause any suffering to an animal, why wouldn't you choose it?"

Indeed. This country goes through a lot of chickens: We raise and kill nearly eight billion a year—about 40 percent of our meat consumption, compared with roughly 30 percent beef and 25 percent pork. Chickens are grown so quickly that *The Veterinary Record* has said that most have bone disease, and many live in chronic pain. (The University of Arkansas reports that if humans grew as fast as chickens, we'd weigh 349 pounds by our second birthday.)

I don't believe chickens have souls, but it's obvious they have real lives, consciousness, and feeling, and they're capable of suffering, so any reduction in the number killed each year would be good.

If that's too touchy-feely for you, how's this? Producers have difficulty efficiently dealing with the manure, wastewater, and post-slaughter residue that result from raising animals industrially; chickens, for example, produce about as much waste as their intake of feed.

Then there's the antibiotic issue: roughly 80 percent of the antibiotics sold in this country are given to animals, which has increased the number of antibiotic-resistant diseases as well as the presence of arsenic in the soil and our food. Work in meat and poultry processing plants is notoriously dangerous. In 2005, Human Rights Watch called it "the most dangerous factory job in America," and nearly every test of supermarket chicken finds high percentages—sometimes as high as two out of three samples—of staph, salmonella, campylobacter, listeria, or the disease-causing antibiotic-resistant bacteria called MRSA. Bill Marler, a leading food safety lawyer, told me he assumes that "almost all chicken and turkey produced in the U.S. is tainted with a bacteria that can kill you."

Until now, cost remained an objection. Some fake meat sells for upward of $12 a pound, which is nearly four times the national average for boneless breasts. Brown says that his price will be below that of chicken.

All of this got me down to Cumberland, Md., where Brown's pilot facility is housed, to make some "chicken" myself. The process mimics that of pasta, breakfast cereal, Cheetos, and, for that matter, plastic. I poured some powder into a hopper—in this instance, soy and pea protein, amaranth, carrot fiber, and a few other ingredients (not many, mostly unobjectionable and of course no antibiotics)—and an extruder mixed it with water, applying various temperatures and pressures to achieve the desired consistency.

The thick strands that emerged on the other end didn't precisely resemble chicken strips, and when I tasted them unadulterated I found it bland, unexciting, and not very chicken-like. But not offensive, either, and as an ingredient we'd all be hard-pressed to distinguish it from most of the animal-based models.

Even the Department of Agriculture is now on the side of plant-based diets. Its "Dietary Guidelines" say "vegetarian-style eating patterns have been associated with improved health outcomes."

And almost all unbiased people agree that less meat is better than more: for our health, for the environment, and certainly for the animals treated as widgets.

MARCH 9, 2012

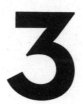

3

What Is Food?
And What Is Not?

Never before in the history of eating has it been harder to make sane food choices. There's a fast-food restaurant on every corner, and a junk food ad on every TV and website. Purportedly "healthy" products like fortified water and granola bars are laced with added sugars (the tobacco of this generation), while actually healthy products like fruits, vegetables, grains, and beans (otherwise known as "real food") are unfairly characterized as unaffordable alternatives to "value" meals. As if that weren't enough, Big Food spends billions of marketing dollars every year to ensure that all of this remains the status quo.

Consequently, cooking has never felt more important than it does now. If you want control of what you eat, if you want to help change the way food is produced, if you want to maximize your health and minimize your impact on the environment in general and climate change in particular, you simply have to cook, for reasons described here.

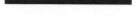

Make Food Choices Simple: Cook

Is there enough food? How do we get it to people? What is its quality? These common questions all concern supply; people spend a lifetime addressing them, and if you closely examine any one, you're ensnared in a complex web.

Yet we don't spend enough time discussing what happens to food once it's in the home. Or what doesn't happen. Which is cooking. And that part is pretty simple.

Not long ago, cooking was a common topic. Weekly food sections of newspapers were filled with it. Churches self-published cookbooks by the pile. There were even real cooking shows and cookbooks.

Now, if it weren't for the vibrant but dwindling community of bloggers, we'd hardly see actual cooking discussed at all. There are but a fraction of the food pages there once were in newspapers, and most cookbooks are offshoots of TV "cooking" shows, almost all of which are game shows, reality television shows, or shows about celebrities.

Like many professional urbanites with grown children, I often succumb to the temptation to work late and eat out with friends. That experience, effortless and pleasurable in anticipation, is usually expensive—even when it's at a theoretically inexpensive restaurant—and frustrating; more often than not it's unsatisfying. (Note that this means it's also sometimes satisfying, which is why I keep doing it; it's a gamble.)

When I cook, though, everything seems to go right. I shop an average of every two weeks in a supermarket, and make a couple of trips a week to smaller stores. I'm aware that my choices are mostly imperfect, but I rarely conclude that I should make a burger and fries for dinner or provide a pound per person of prison-raised pork served with fruit from 10,000 miles away, followed by a cake full of sugar and artificial ingredients. Yet, for the most part, that describes restaurant food.

In the summer, I'll buy local greens and local fish and wind up eating half or less of the food I would have if I had eaten out. Dessert only happens if someone else buys or makes it because I won't do either; I might schlep home a piece of watermelon. The starter, if there is one, might range from bread with butter or oil to homemade hummus or other bean dip to home-roasted or fried nuts, or some salami or ham, hunks of which remain in the fridge for weeks.

That's pretty much it. The investment is minimal: A quick shopping trip takes me a half-hour, including the walk or drive. It takes me about half or three-quarters of an hour to cook, not including the time that it took to make that bean dip or bread, both of which last for days. The time spent eating is relaxing and uninterrupted by the insipid ritual: "Is everything tasting to your liking?" or "You guys O.K.?" It takes 10 minutes to clean up.

Compared with a restaurant, the frustrations and annoyances are minimal, the food is as good or better-tasting, unquestionably healthier and more environmentally friendly, and much less expensive. Saturday night, for example, I fed four people a dinner of nuts, a small frittata, fish, salad, and watermelon for far less than two of us would have spent at Applebee's.

It's not that I'm unconcerned about the supply side. I can't help bugging myself with questions about whether the food I buy is "good" enough: pesticides? fertilizer? endangered fish? carbon footprint? fair pay for farmworkers?

But these are shopping questions, not cooking and eating questions. Shopping is the time to be critical. (Eating is the time to enjoy.) Buy things that you feel answer to your standards, and you'll be a cut above most restaurant food in every category. You'll know exactly what you're putting in your mouth and how much of it. (Who buys 20-ounce steaks for one person at home?) You'll move in the right direction, cooking and eating less meat and junk and more plants.

In most restaurants, the questions are pointless because you relinquish all control. At McDonald's, the main goals seem to involve making the food safe and consistent, not producing it ethically. (They would surely argue with this, and, perhaps, they've made some progress. But really?) In pricier restaurants, the goal seems to be to impress you with presentation, originality, and glamour.

I recognize that I'm privileged, though, in fact, I have friends who are better cooks than I am, who have access to better food and who have more leisure.

I recognize, too, that there are many people for whom time and money and skills and even access are challenges. The thing, though, is not to discount this argument simply because not everyone is in a position to benefit from it, but rather to use it to benefit those it can, and to create the same possibilities for everyone.

JULY 2, 2011

Is Junk Food Really Cheaper?

The "fact" that junk food is cheaper than real food has become a reflexive part of how we explain why so many Americans are overweight, particularly those with lower incomes. I frequently read confident statements like, "when a bag of chips is cheaper than a head of broccoli . . ." or "it's more affordable to feed a family of four at McDonald's than to cook a healthy meal for them at home."

This is just plain wrong. In fact it isn't cheaper to eat highly processed food: a typical order for a family of four—for example, two Big Macs, a cheeseburger, six chicken McNuggets, two medium and two small fries, and two medium and two small sodas—costs, at the McDonald's a hundred steps from where I write, about $28. (Judicious ordering of "Happy Meals" can reduce that to about $23—and you get a few apple slices in addition to the fries!)

In general, despite extensive government subsidies, hyperprocessed food remains more expensive than food cooked at home. You can serve a roasted chicken with vegetables along with a simple salad and milk for about $14, and feed four or even six people. If that's too much money, substitute a meal of rice and canned beans with bacon, green peppers, and onions; it's easily enough for four people and costs about $9. (Omitting the bacon, using dried beans, which are also lower in sodium, or substituting carrots for the peppers reduces the price even further.)

Another argument runs that junk food is cheaper when measured by the calorie, and that this makes fast food essential for the poor because they need cheap calories. But given that half of the people in this country (and a higher percentage of poor people) consume too many calories rather than too few, measuring food's value by the calorie makes as much sense as measuring a drink's value by its alcohol content. (Why not drink 95 percent neutral grain spirit, the cheapest way to get drunk?)

Besides, that argument, even if we all needed to gain weight, is not always true. A meal of real food cooked at home can easily contain more calories, most of them of the "healthy" variety. (Olive oil accounts for many of the calories in the roast chicken meal, for example.) In comparing prices of real food and junk food, I used supermarket ingredients, not the pricier organic or local food that many people would consider ideal. But food choices are not black and white; the alternative to fast food is not necessarily organic food, any more than the alternative to soda is Bordeaux.

The alternative to soda is water, and the alternative to junk food is not grass-fed beef and greens from a trendy farmers' market, but anything other than junk food: rice, grains, pasta, beans, fresh vegetables, canned vegetables, frozen vegetables, meat, fish, poultry, dairy products, bread, peanut butter, a thousand other things cooked at home—in almost every case a far superior alternative.

"Anything that you do that's not fast food is terrific; cooking once a week is far better than not cooking at all," says Marion Nestle, professor of food studies at New York University and author of *What to Eat*. "It's the same argument as exercise: more is better than less and some is a lot better than none."

The fact is that most people *can* afford real food. Even the nearly 50 million Americans who are enrolled in the Supplemental Nutrition Assistance Program (formerly known as food stamps) receive about $5 per person per day, which is far from ideal but enough to survive. So we have to assume that money alone doesn't guide decisions about what to eat. There are, of course, the so-called food deserts, places where it's hard to find food: the Department of Agriculture says that more than two million Americans in low-income rural areas live 10 miles or more from a supermarket, and more than five million households without access to cars live more than a half mile from a supermarket.

Still, 93 percent of those with limited access to supermarkets do have access to vehicles, though it takes them 20 more minutes to travel to the store than the national average. And after a long day of work at one or even two jobs, 20 extra minutes—plus cooking time—must seem like an eternity.

Taking the long route to putting food on the table may not be easy, but for almost all Americans it remains a choice, and if you can drive to McDonald's you can drive to Safeway. It's cooking that's the real challenge. (The real challenge is not "I'm too busy to cook." In 2010 the average American, regardless of weekly earnings, watched no less than an hour and a half of television per day. The time is there.)

The core problem is that cooking is defined as work, and fast food is both a pleasure and a crutch. "People really are stressed out with all that they have to do, and they don't want to cook," says Julie Guthman, associate professor of community studies at the University of California, Santa Cruz, and author of the forthcoming *Weighing In: Obesity, Food Justice and the Limits of Capitalism.* "Their reaction is, 'Let me enjoy what I want to eat, and stop telling me what to do.' And it's one of the few things that less well-off people have: they don't have to cook."

It's not just about choice, however, and rational arguments go only so far, because money and access and time and skill are not the only considerations. The ubiquity, convenience and habit-forming appeal of hyperprocessed foods have largely drowned out the alternatives: there are five fast-food restaurants for every supermarket in the United States; in recent decades the adjusted for inflation price of fresh produce has increased by 40 percent while the price of soda and processed food has decreased by as much as 30 percent; and nearly inconceivable resources go into encouraging consumption in restaurants: fast-food companies spent $4.2 billion on marketing in 2009.

Furthermore, the engineering behind hyperprocessed food makes it virtually addictive. A 2009 study by the Scripps Research Institute indicates that overconsumption of fast food "triggers addiction-like neuroaddictive responses" in the brain, making it harder to trigger the release of dopamine. In other words the more fast food we eat, the more we need to give us pleasure; thus the report suggests that the same mechanisms underlie drug addiction and obesity.

This addiction to processed food is the result of decades of vision and hard work by the industry. For 50 years, says David A. Kessler, former commissioner of the Food and Drug Administration and author of *The End of Overeating,* companies strove to create food that was "energy-dense, highly stimulating, and went down easy. They put it on every street corner and made it mobile, and they made it socially acceptable to eat anytime and anyplace. They created a food carnival, and that's where we live. And if you're used to self-stimulation every 15 minutes, well, you can't run into the kitchen to satisfy that urge."

Real cultural changes are needed to turn this around. Somehow, no-nonsense cooking and eating—roasting a chicken, making a grilled cheese sandwich, scrambling an egg, tossing a salad—must become popular again, and valued not just by hipsters in Brooklyn or locavores in Berkeley. The smart campaign is not to get McDonald's to serve better food but to get people to see cooking as a joy rather than a burden, or at least as part of a normal life.

As with any addictive behavior, this one is most easily countered by educating children about the better way. Children, after all, are born without bad habits. And yet it's adults who must begin to tear down the food carnival.

The question is how. Efforts are everywhere. The People's Grocery in Oakland secures affordable groceries for low-income people. Zoning laws in Los Angeles restrict the number of fast-food restaurants in high-obesity neighborhoods. There's the Healthy Food Financing Initiative, a successful Pennsylvania program to build fresh food outlets in underserved areas, now being expanded nationally. FoodCorps and Cooking Matters teach young people how to farm and cook.

As Malik Yakini, executive director of the Detroit Black Community Food Security Network, says, "We've seen minor successes, but the food movement is still at the infant stage, and we need a massive social shift to convince people to consider healthier options."

How do you change a culture? The answers, not surprisingly, are complex. "Once I look at what I'm eating," says Dr. Kessler, "and realize it's not food, and I ask 'what am I doing here?' that's the start. It's not about whether I think it's good for me, it's about changing how I feel. And we change how people feel by changing the environment."

Obviously, in an atmosphere where any regulation is immediately labeled "nanny-statism," changing "the environment" is difficult. But we've done this before, with tobacco. The 1998 tobacco settlement limited cigarette marketing and forced manufacturers to finance anti-smoking campaigns—a negotiated change that led to an environmental one that in turn led to a cultural one, after which kids said to their parents, "I wish you didn't smoke." Smoking had to be converted from a cool habit into one practiced by pariahs.

A similar victory in the food world is symbolized by the stories parents tell me of their kids booing as they drive by McDonald's.

To make changes like this more widespread we need action both cultural and political. The cultural lies in celebrating real food; raising our children in homes that don't program them for fast-produced, eaten-on-the-run, high-calorie, low-nutrition junk; giving them the gift of appreciating the pleasures of nourishing one another and enjoying that nourishment together.

Political action would mean agitating to limit the marketing of junk; forcing its makers to pay the true costs of production; recognizing that advertising for fast food is not the exercise of free speech but behavior manipulation of addictive substances; and making certain that real food is affordable and available to everyone. The political challenge is the more difficult one, but it cannot be ignored.

What's easier is to cook at every opportunity, to demonstrate to family and neighbors that the real way is the better way. And even the more fun way: kind of like a carnival.

AUGUST 25, 2011

What Is Food?

If you believe government has no role in helping people—including encouraging us to act in our own best interests by doing things like not smoking, wearing seat belts, and getting exercise—you're probably no fan of New York's mayor, Michael R. Bloomberg. The mayor, who has already banned smoking in bars and trans fats from restaurant food, has created more bike lanes in his administration than all other administrations combined and forced the posting of calorie counts in fast-food restaurants, added to his sins by proposing a ban on the sale of sugar-sweetened beverages (SSBs) over one pint (16 ounces) in a variety of venues.

The arguments against this ban mostly come from the "right." (There actually is no right and left here, only right and wrong.) We're told, as we almost always are when a progressive public health measure is passed, that this is "nanny-statism." (The American Beverage Association also argues that the move is counterproductive, but the cigarette companies used to market their product as healthful, so as long as you remember that, you know what to do with the A.B.A.'s statements.) On a more personal level, we hear things like, "if people want to be obese, that's their prerogative."

Certainly. And if people want to ride motorcycles without helmets or smoke cigarettes that's their prerogative, too. But it's the nanny-state's prerogative to protect the rest of us from their idiotic behavior. Sugar-sweetened beverages account for a full 7 percent of our calorie intake, and those calories are not just "empty," as is often said, but harmful: obesity-related health care costs are at $147 billion and climbing.

To (loosely) paraphrase Oliver Wendell Holmes, your right to harm yourself stops when I have to pay for it. And just as we all pay for the ravages of smoking, we all pay for the harmful effects of Coke, Snapple, and Gatorade.

Let's be clear: Sugar-sweetened beverages are nothing more than sugar delivery systems, and sugar is probably the most dangerous part of our current diet. People will argue forever about whether sugar-sweetened beverages lead directly to obesity, but Bloomberg's ban should be framed first and foremost as an effort to reduce sugar consumption. Good.

Some have criticized the mayor's step as weak. But his public health staff, led by the estimable health commissioner, Thomas A. Farley, has already tried to pass a tax on soda (unquestionably the most effective tool in our box to reduce the consumption of sugar-sweetened beverages) but were rebuffed by Albany. They've also tried to prohibit the use of food stamps through the Supplemental Nutrition Assistance Program, or SNAP, to buy soda, and been rebuffed—lamely—by the Department of Agriculture's secretary, Tom Vilsack. (Food stamps are currently used to purchase billions worth of soda a year, a nice subsidy for soda and commodity corn producers, as well as for makers of insulin.)

Was this the mayor's optimal move? I asked Farley that question. His response: "This is the best way to go to have a substantial influence on portion size right now, and people still have the freedom to continue to buy sugar-sweetened beverages," thereby throwing a bone to those who evidently believe that it's impossible to sit through a ballgame or a movie without at least a quart of Mountain Dew.

If the mayor were to ban 32-ounce mugs of beer at Yankee Stadium after a number of D.U.I. arrests—and, indeed, there are limits to drinking at ballparks—we would not be hearing about his nanny tendencies. (And certainly most non-smokers, at least, are ecstatic that smoking in public places— including Central Park—is increasingly forbidden.) No one questions the prohibition on the use of SNAP for tobacco and alcohol. And that's because we accept that these things are not food.

So perhaps we ask: What, exactly, is food? My dictionary calls it "any nutritious substance that people or animals eat or drink, or that plants absorb, in order to maintain life and growth." That doesn't help so much unless you define nutritious. Nutritious food, it says here, "provides those substances necessary for growth, health, and good condition."

Sugar-sweetened beverages don't meet this description any more than do beer and tobacco and, for that matter, heroin, and they have more in common with these things than they do with carrots. They promote growth all right—in precisely the wrong way—and they do the opposite of promoting health and good condition. They are not food.

Added sugar, as will be obvious when we look back in 20 or 50 years, is the tobacco of the 21st century. (The time frame will depend on how many decent public health officials we manage to put in office, and how hard we're willing to fight Big Food.) And if you believe that limiting our "right" to purchase soda is a slippery slope, one that will lead to defining which foods are nutritious and which aren't—and which ones government funds should be used to subsidize and which they shouldn't—you're right. It's the beginning of better public health policy, policy that is good for the health of our citizenry.

We should be encouraging people to eat real food and discouraging the consumption of non-food. Pretending there's no difference is siding with the merchants of death who would have us eat junk at the expense of food and spend half our lives earning enough money to deal with the health consequences.

Right now a tall 5-year-old with a dollar can approach a machine and buy a fizzy beverage equivalent to a cup of coffee with nine teaspoons of sugar in it. And that's a mere 12 ounces. Holding the line at that seems to make some sense. Unless you somehow define harmful, non-food substances as something other than "bad."

JUNE 5, 2012

Is "Eat Real Food" Unthinkable?

In recent weeks we've seen a big, powerful government agency, a big, powerful person, and a big, powerful corporation telling us what to eat. Even with all this big, powerful input, we know nothing that we didn't know last year. We do, however, have a new acronym; unfortunately, it's not the one we need.

And a little progress. Limited kudos go to the United States Department of Agriculture, whose Dietary Guidelines for Americans, 2010—yes, it's 2011, but they're published every five years—are the best to date. We're told to eat "less food" and more fresh foods; wise advice. But aside from salt, the agency buries mostly vague recommendations about what we should be eating less of: we're admonished to consume "few or no" sodas—hooray for that—and "refined grains," Solid Fats and Added Sugars. And there's our fabulous acronym: SOFAS.

The problem, as usual, is that the agency's nutrition experts are at odds with its other mission: to promote our bounty in whatever form its processors make it. The U.S.D.A. can succeed at its conflicting goals only by convincing us that eating manufactured food lower in SOFAS is "healthy," thus implicitly endorsing hyper-engineered junk food with added fiber, reduced solid fats, and so on, "food" that is often unimaginably far from its origins. When it comes to eating more "good" food, the report is clear, because that can't harm producers. When it comes to eating less of what's "bad," the language turns to "science," because telling us which products to avoid—like a 3,000-calorie fast-food "meal" or a box of low-fat but chemical-laden crackers—would play badly with industry. Instead we're told to avoid SOFAS. Where's that SOFAS aisle?

The report might have led with Michael Pollan's ground-breaking slogan—"Eat food. Not too much. Mostly plants."—and then explained details in a few pages. But although the agency's advisory committee suggested a "shift . . . toward a more plant-based diet," the report itself backs "a healthy eating pattern," and then, over 100-plus pages, is largely imprecise, probably to avoid offending meat and sugar lobbies. (The salt lobby is evidently puny.)

In its attempts to upset no one powerful, the U.S.D.A. offers a typically contorted message. The advice people need is to cook and eat more real food, at the expense of the junk served in most restaurants and take-out places. In fact, most of the mysterious SOFAS come from so-called "fast" and "convenient" food, as does most sodium. (The salt shaker is not the culprit.)

It isn't easy to cook with the junk that makes junk food junky, but the agency spends little energy boosting cooking. There is the, "Cook and eat more meals at home . . . include vegetables, fruits, whole grains, fat-free or low-fat dairy products, and protein foods that provide fewer calories and more nutrients." But it stands almost alone, and could have been far simpler and stronger. Why isn't it? Because "protein foods that provide fewer calories" doesn't offend the meat industry, as Pollan's motto does.

Which brings us to the powerful person: Oprah. Ms. Winfrey, who has been on more diets than the rest of us combined, challenged her staff to "go vegan" for a week. Intriguing, except her idea of surviving without meat and dairy—no explanation given for why we should go from too much to none—is to fill your shopping cart with fake versions of both, like meatless chicken breasts and dairy-less cheese.

But the goal is not universal veganism, which is pie-in-the-sky; it's health and sustainability. And we get there by preparing real food, vegan or not. (Remember: Coke, Tostitos, and Reese's Peanut Butter Puffs—yum!—are all vegan.) The answer is not fake animal products, whose advocates argue that they're transitional to a kinder-to-animal diet. Indeed, that's good, but a real food diet is better.

Finally, our powerful corporation—Walmart—whose alliance with Michelle Obama looks pretty good, at least at first. We are promised more affordable produce, which undoubtedly means that Walmart will beat the living daylights out of produce suppliers, crushing a few thousand more small farmers. (In fact, what we need is higher-quality and probably more expensive produce, that which is less damaging to the environment, laborers, and consumers, but that gets into the "how do we afford it?" argument, which must wait for another day. Let's leave it that we like Walmart's goal of selling more produce.)

The real problem, again, is Walmart's other promise: "healthier" pack-aged foods. And whether baked, low-salt chips are "better" than fried ones is not only arguable—the baked ones are more likely to be chemical-laden—but misses the point, which, again, is that real foods are superior in every way.

The truly healthy alternative to that chip is not a fake chip; it's a carrot. Likewise, the alternative to sausage is not vegan sausage; it's less sausage. This is really all pretty simple, and pretty clear. But the messages we've heard re-cently are as clear as . . . well, a SOFA.

You want an acronym? Let's try ERF: Eat Real Food.

FEBRUARY 8, 2011

Why Won't McDonald's Really Lead?

Every McDonald's executive I've met who happens to be a parent says something like this: "I don't let my kids eat at McDonald's all the time. It's a treat; we know that." Yet these same executives, in literature and in public, say that they're "championing children's well-being."

Big Mac is confused. It remains among the world's most envied brands, yet its unique position means it must—or at least should—lead within the industry. But despite the company's claims, its tardiness in marketing real, healthful food solidifies Big Mac's public image as a pusher and profiteer of junk food, incapable of doing (or unwilling to do) the right thing. Envied by the competition, beloved by at least some customers, McDonald's is reviled by those who see it as setting undesirable eating patterns in children, patterns that remain for life.

Despite the fact that the company removed images of soda from national advertising for its Happy Meals, it comprises 57 percent of the beverages sold to kids. And, despite a well-publicized announcement in which the company promised to market only water, milk, and juice in its Happy Meal advertising, there's little sign of the sugar-peddling diminishing. It's true that 21 percent of all Happy Meals are now sold with milk, but the vast majority of that is chocolate milk, which, according to the company's fascinating nutrition charts (you should look), contains about 10 grams of added sugar per serving, about the same as you'd get in 20 M&Ms. This is progress?

Yet McDonald's is as good a spinmaster as any. (They're like Speaker Boehner: in the history books already, but still with a chance to influence the reason.) Thus the company and some surprising allies descended on New York with yet another announcement about its "healthier" food.

The news was developed in conjunction with the Alliance for a Healthier Generation (what were they thinking?), a joint venture of the Clinton Global Initiative and the American Heart Association. And although it would have been fun to see the former president preach his part-time veganism to his McDonald's partners—Hey guys! How about a Meatless Monday?—instead we found Big Bill less critical of McDonald's than he was of welfare. We learned mostly that the company will "increase customers' access to fruit and vegetables and help families and children to make informed choices in keeping with balanced lifestyles." You can imagine.

First McDonald's promised that it would no longer "promote and market" soda in Happy Meals; only time will tell if that's the precise truth. This means, according to a spokeswoman, that within five years, "sodas will no longer be listed on the Happy Meal menu boards in the specified 20 major markets that represent 85% of our global sales."

It doesn't mean you'll be asked only whether your kid prefers milk, water, or juice; it just means there won't be pictures of soda with Happy Meals on the menu boards. It's not like milk will become the default. No: McDonald's will actively discourage the drinking of soda (likely its most profitable item and among the least healthy items in the American diet) only when it's forced to.

The company also pledges to offer fruit, a vegetable, or a salad with so-called Value Meals for those customers who would prefer one of those instead of fries. You could say this would expand choice, and you'd be right; it's not a complete failure. But as they say, no one goes into McDonald's looking for salad.

McDonald's and its brethren want some love; they want people like Marion Nestle, Michele Simon, and me to stop kvetching and instead acknowledge that they're making great strides in promoting health rather than "illth" . . . but only the most gullible buy that.

For example. The company boasts of having served 440 million cups of fruits and vegetables to its customers between mid-2012 and mid-2013. But let's do some math: McDonald's serves 28,000,000 people a day, which translates to around 10 billion customers a year. So those 440 million cups? That's only about .04 cups more per customer, per day. Compare this to something like a billion pounds of beef.

I used to joke that many Americans counted the lettuce on a hamburger as a serving of vegetables. But it's not a leaf of lettuce: it's a shred. It would appear that McDonald's idea of "bold nutrition moves" (a phrase used by McDonald's senior vice president Greg Watson) is a shred of lettuce.

The timetable for even these modest changes—which, for all we know, will preclude any meaningful changes during the phase-in period—is laughable: it will take place in 30 to 50 percent of 20 major markets within three years and the remainder of those markets by 2020. So in seven years most McDonald's customers a) won't have soda forced upon them and b) will, upon request, be able to not have fries with that.

McDonald's thinks its customers are afraid of change, and it may be right; but it's in a bind. The company is already failing with the coveted millennials market and may even be losing steam when it comes to kids. A bold marketing move would see real food and real health as a huge opportunity in fast food, and the dozens of successful new companies that do so are starting to eat McDonald's lunch.

But although Mr. Watson told me that at any given time there are "around 50" new products being tested in the Mickey D pipeline, the company is afraid that its customers "just aren't ready" for something like a veggie burger. They say things like, "You told us you're trying harder to be more nutrition-minded for yourself and for your family. We listened." But what they do is introduce McWraps—many of which have unfavorable nutrition profiles even when compared to burgers—and make it marginally easier for the best-educated, most assertive of their customers to demand marginally better choices.

If McDonald's wanted to be on the right side of history, it would announce something like this: "Starting tomorrow, we're not offering soda with Happy Meals except by specific request. And starting Jan. 1, at every McDonald's, we'll be offering a small burger with a big salad for the price of a burger and fries to anyone who asks for it; we're also adding a chopped salad McWrap. We challenge our competitors to follow us in making fast food as healthful as it is affordable, and we dare our critics to say we're not changing."

That ain't gonna happen. But if it did, I'd be the first in line to applaud.

OCTOBER 8, 2013

Parasites, Killing Their Host

The Food Industry's Solution to Obesity

You can buy food from farmers—directly, through markets, any way you can find—and I hope you do. But unless you're radically different from most of us, much of what you eat comes from corporations that process, market, deliver, and sell "food," a majority of which is processed beyond recognition.

The problem is that real food isn't real profitable. "It's hard to market fruit and vegetables without adding value," says Marion Nestle, a professor of nutrition, food studies, and public health at New York University. "If you turn a potato into a potato chip you not only make more money—you create a product with a long shelf life." Potatoes into chips and frozen fries; wheat into soft, "enriched" bread; soybeans into oil and meat; corn into meat and a staggering variety of junk.

How do we break this cycle? You can't blame corporations for trying to profit by any means necessary, even immoral ones: It's their nature.

You can possibly blame them for stupidity: Even a mindless parasite knows that if it kills its host the party's over, and by pushing products that promote "illth"—the opposite of health—Big Food is unwittingly destroying its own market. Diet-related Type 2 diabetes and cardiovascular disease disable and kill people, and undoubtedly we'll be hearing more about nonalcoholic steatohepatitis, or NASH, an increasingly prevalent fatty liver disease that's brought on by diet and may lead to liver failure.

Food companies are well aware of the health crisis their products cause, and recognize that the situation is unsustainable. But one theory has it that as long as even one of the big food companies remains cynical and uncaring about its market, they all must remain so.

Chief among the hopeful arguments is one that goes something like this: The first big food outfit to recognize that its future lies in creating a market for healthy and even environmentally neutral food (let's throw in justice for workers and animal welfare while we're at it!) may show the way to the future of healthy food as a sound business model. Some profitable corporations nibble at the edges of this already, but—as a piece in the current *Harvard Business Review* points out—American capitalists have become poor innovators.

Only the naïve, however, would believe that Big Food is generally working toward this. As Nestle and Michele Simon, author of *Appetite for Profit,* have been saying for years, these organizations represent not the public interest but the corporate one, and since they haven't devised a way to improve or even maintain their bottom lines selling real food, they have to appear to be selling "better" food.

But the key remains selling. A new paper in the journal *Social Currents* by Ivy Ken, an associate professor of sociology at George Washington University, discusses Big Food's strategy of "working together" with communities to fight the obesity crisis. The goal is threefold, according to Ken: Corporations want us to focus on the importance of their role in "solving" childhood obesity and presenting themselves as part of the solution. "Their part of working together is re-engineering their products; our part of working together is to buy more and more of this food that's not real," Ken said to me.

The food industry also wants us to ignore its use of that strategy to increase its market share and profits; and it wants to maintain legitimacy at a time when community groups and public health officials are, writes Ken, "demanding limits to their involvement" in supplying food to children.

Our efforts to demand limits on the sale of junk to children are a threat to Big Food. If we succeed, it fails, or at least suffers. But if industry succeeds, whether in selling blatant junk or re-engineered versions that are low in fat or sodium (or gluten or sugar-free or reduced-calorie or high fiber or whatever—companies can create any frankenfood they feel will sell), we will continue to suffer. (Nestle often says, "A slightly-better-for-you junk food is still junk food.") Our health will decline further, the environment will be further degraded, and our health care system (and therefore economy) will spend an increasingly disproportionate amount of money on diet-generated chronic disease.

If the most profitable scenario means that most food choices are essentially toxic—in the sense that overconsumption will cause illness—that's a failure of the market, not of individual choice. And government's rightful role is not to form partnerships with industry so that the latter can voluntarily "solve" the problem, but to oversee and regulate industry. Its mandate is to protect public health, and one good step toward fulfilling that right now would be to regulate the marketing of junk to children. Anything short of that is a failure.

JUNE 17, 2014

Yes, Healthful Fast Food Is Possible. But Edible?

When my daughter was a teenager, about a dozen years ago, she went through a vegetarian phase. Back then, the payoff for orthodontist visits was a trip to Taco Bell, where the only thing we could eat were bean burritos and tacos. It wasn't my favorite meal, but the mushy beans in that soft tortilla or crisp shell were kind of soothing, and the sweet "hot" sauce made the experience decent enough. I usually polished off two or three.

I was thinking of those Taco Bell stops during a recent week of travel. I had determined, as a way of avoiding the pitfalls of airport food, to be vegan for the length of the trip. This isn't easy. By the time I got to Terminal C at Dallas/Fort Worth, I couldn't bear another Veggie Delite from Subway, a bad chopped salad on lousy bread. So I wandered up to the Taco Bell Express opposite Gate 14 and optimistically asked the cashier if I could get a bean burrito without cheese or sour cream. He pointed out a corner on the overhead display where the "fresco" menu offered pico de gallo in place of dairy, then upsold me on a multilayered "fresco" bean burrito for about 3 bucks. As he was talking, the customers to my right and left, both fit, suit-wearing people bearing expressions of hunger and resignation, perked up. They weren't aware of the fresco menu, either. One was trying to "eat healthy on the road"; the other copped to "having vegan kids." Like me, they were intrigued by a fast-food burrito with about 350 calories, or less than half as many as a Fiesta Taco Salad bowl. It wasn't bad, either.

Twelve years after the publication of *Fast Food Nation* and nearly as long since Morgan Spurlock almost ate himself to death, our relationship with fast food has changed. We've gone from the whistle-blowing stage to the higher-expectations stage, and some of those expectations are being met. Various states have passed measures to limit the confinement of farm animals. In-N-Out Burger has demonstrated that you don't have to underpay your employees to be profitable. There are dozens of plant-based alternatives to meat, with more on the way; increasingly, they're pretty good.

The fulfillment of these expectations has led to higher ones. My experience at the airport only confirmed what I'd been hearing for years from analysts in the fast-food industry. After the success of companies like Whole Foods, and healthful (or theoretically healthful) brands like Annie's and Kashi, there's now a market for a fast-food chain that's not only healthful itself, but vegetarian-friendly, sustainable, and even humane. And, this being fast food: cheap. "It is significant, and I do believe it is coming from consumer desire to have choices and more balance," says Andy Barish, a restaurant analyst at Jefferies LLC, the investment bank. "And it's not just the coasts anymore."

I'm not talking about token gestures, like McDonald's fruit-and-yogurt parfait, whose calories are more than 50 percent sugar. And I don't expect the prices to match those of Taco Bell or McDonald's, where economies of scale and inexpensive ingredients make meals dirt cheap. What I'd like is a place that serves only good options, where you don't have to resist the junk food to order well, and where the food is real—by which I mean dishes that generally contain few ingredients and are recognizable to everyone, not just food technologists. It's a place where something like a black-bean burger piled with vegetables and baked sweet potato fries—and, hell, maybe even a vegan shake—is less than 10 bucks and 800 calories (and way fewer without the shake). If I could order and eat that in 15 minutes, I'd be happy, and I think a lot of others would be, too. You can try my recipes for a fast, low-calorie burger, fries, and shake.

In recent years, the fast-food industry has started to heed these new demands. Billions of dollars have been invested in more healthful fast-food options, and the financial incentives justify these expenditures. About half of all the money spent on food in the United States is for meals eaten outside the home. And last year McDonald's earned $5.5 billion in profits on $88 billion in sales. If a competitor offered a more healthful option that was able to capture just a single percent of that market share, it would make $55 million. Chipotle, the best newcomer of the last generation, has beaten that 1 percent handily. Last year, sales approached $3 billion. In the fourth quarter, they grew by 17 percent over the same period in the previous year.

Numbers are tricky to pin down for more healthful options because the fast-food industry doesn't yet have a category for "healthful." The industry re-fers to McDonald's and Burger King as "quick-serve restaurants"; Chipotle is "fast casual"; and restaurants where you order at the counter and the food is brought to you are sometimes called "premium fast casual." Restaurants from these various sectors often deny these distinctions, but *QSR*, an industry trade magazine—"Limited-Service, Unlimited Possibilities"—spends a good deal of space dissecting them.

However, after decades of eating the stuff, I have my own. First, there are those places that serve junk, no matter what kind of veneer they present. Sub-way, Taco Bell (I may be partial to them, but really . . .), McDonald's, and their ilk make up the Junk Food sector. One step up are places with better ambi-ence and perhaps better ingredients—Shake Shack, Five Guys, Starbucks, Pret a Manger—that also peddle unhealthful food but succeed in making diners feel better about eating it, either because it tastes better, is surrounded by some healthful options, the setting is groovier, or they use some organic or sustain-able ingredients. This is the Nouveau Junk sector.

Chipotle combines the best aspects of Nouveau Junk to create a new cat-egory that we might call Improved Fast Food. At Chipotle, the food is fresher and tastes much better than traditional fast food. The sourcing, production, and cooking is generally of a higher level; and the overall experience is more pleasant. The guacamole really is made on premises, and the chicken (however tasteless) is cooked before your eyes. It's fairly easy to eat vegan there, but those burritos can pack on the calories. As a competitor told me, "Several brands had a head start on [the Chipotle founder Steve] Ells, but he kicked their [expletive] with culture and quality. It's not shabby for assembly-line steam-table Mexican food. It might be worth $10 billion right now." (It is.)

Chipotle no longer stands alone in the Improved Fast Food world: Chop't, Maoz, Freshii, Zoës Kitchen, and several others all have their strong points. And—like Chipotle—they all have their limitations, starting with calories and fat. By offering fried chicken and fried onions in addition to organic tofu, Chop't, a salad chain in New York and Washington, tempts customers to turn what might have been a healthful meal into a calorie bomb (to say nothing of the tasteless dressing), and often raises the price to $12 or more. The Netherlands-based Maoz isn't bad, but it's not as good as the mom-and-pop falafel trucks and shops that are all over Manhattan. There are barely any choices, nothing is cooked to order, the pita is a sponge, and there is a messy serve-yourself setup that makes a $10 meal seem like a bit of a rip-off.

Despite its flaws, Improved Fast Food is the transitional step to a new category of fast-food restaurant whose practices should be even closer to sustainable and whose meals should be reasonably healthful and good-tasting and inexpensive. (Maybe not McDonald's-inexpensive, but under $10.) This new category is, or will be, Good Fast Food, and there are already a few emerging contenders.

Veggie Grill is a six-year-old Los Angeles–based chain with 18 locations. Technically, it falls into the "premium fast casual" category. The restaurants are pleasantly designed and nicely lighted and offer limited service. The food is strictly vegan, though you might not know it at first.

Kevin Boylan and T. K. Pillan, the chain's founders, are vegans themselves. They frequently refer to their food as "familiar" and "American," but that's debatable. The "chickin" in the "Santa Fe Crispy Chickin" sandwich is Gardein, a soy-based product that has become the default for fast-food operators looking for meat substitutes. Although there are better products in the pipeline, Gardein, especially when fried, tastes more or less like a McNugget (which isn't entirely "real" chicken itself). The "cheese" is Daiya, which is tapioca-based and similar in taste to a pasteurized processed American cheese. The "steak," "carne asada," "crab cake" (my favorite), and "burger" are also soy, in combination with wheat and pea protein. In terms of animal welfare, environmental damage, and resource usage, these products are huge steps in the right direction. They save animals, water, energy, and land.

Boylan wanted to make clear to me that his chain isn't about haute cuisine. "We're not doing sautéed tempeh with a peach reduction da-da-da," he said. "That may be a great menu item, but most people don't know what it is. When we say 'cheeseburger'—or 'fried chickin' with mashed potatoes with gravy and steamed kale—everyone knows what we're talking about." He's probably right, and the vegetables are pretty good, too. The mashed potatoes are cut with 40 percent cauliflower; the gravy is made from porcini mushrooms and you can get your entree on a bed of kale instead of a bun.

When I first entered a Veggie Grill, I expected a room full of skinny vegans talking about their vegan-ness. Instead, at locations in Hollywood, El Segundo, and Westwood, the lines could have been anywhere, even an airport Taco Bell. The diners appeared mixed by class and weight, and sure looked like omnivores, which they mostly are. The company's research shows that about 70 percent of its customers eat meat or fish, a fact that seems both reflected in its menu and its instant success. Veggie Grill won best American restaurant in the 2012 *Los*

Angeles Times readers' poll, and sales are up 16 percent in existing stores compared with last year. The plan is to double those 18 locations every 18 months for the foreseeable future—"fast enough to stay ahead of competitors, but not so fast as to lose our cultural DNA," Boylan said. In 2011, the founders brought in a new C.E.O., Greg Dollarhyde, who helped Baja Fresh become a national chain before its sale to Wendy's for nearly $300 million.

Veggie Grill is being underwritten partly by Brentwood Associates, a small private-equity firm that's invested in various consumer businesses, including Zoës Kitchen, a chain that offers kebabs, braised beans, and roasted vegetables. "For a firm like us to get involved with a concept like Veggie Grill, we have to believe it's a profitable business model, and we do," Brentwood's managing director, Rahul Aggarwal, told me. "Ten years ago I would've said no vegan restaurant would be successful, but people are looking for different ways to eat and this is a great concept."

I admire Veggie Grill, but while making "chickin" from soy is no crime, it's still far from real food. I have a long-running argument with committed vegan friends, who say that Americans aren't ready for rice and beans, or chickpea-and-spinach stew, and that places like Veggie Grill offer a transition to animal-and-environment-friendlier food. On one level, I agree. Why feed the grain to tortured animals to produce lousy meat when you can process the grain and produce it into "meat"? On another level, the goal should be fast food that's real food, too.

Much of what I ate at Veggie Grill was fried and dense, and even when I didn't overeat, I felt as heavy afterward as I do after eating at a Junk Food chain. And while that Santa Fe Crispy Chickin sandwich with lettuce, tomato, red onion, avocado, and vegan mayo comes in at 550 calories, 200 fewer than Burger King's Tendercrisp chicken sandwich, the "chickin" sandwich costs $9. The Tendercrisp costs $5, and that's in Midtown Manhattan.

Future growth should allow Veggie Grill to lower prices, but it may never be possible to spend less than 10 dollars on a meal there. Part of that cost is service: at Veggie Grill, you order, get a number to put on your table, and wait for a server. It's a luxury compared with most chains, and a pleasant one, but the combination of the food's being not quite real and the price's being still too high means Veggie Grill hasn't made the leap to Good Fast Food.

During my time in Los Angeles, I also ate at Native Foods Café, a vegan chain similar to Veggie Grill, where you can get a pretty good "meatball" sub (made of seitan, a form of wheat gluten), and at Tender Greens, which, though it is cafeteria-style (think Chipotle with a large Euro-Californian menu), flirts with the $20 mark for a meal. It can't really be considered fast food, but it's quite terrific and I'd love to see it put Applebee's and Olive Garden out of business.

In Culver City, I visited Lyfe Kitchen (that's "Love Your Food Everyday"; I know, but please keep reading). Lyfe has the pedigree, menu, financing, plan, and ambition to take on the major chains. The company is trying to build 250 locations in the next five years, and QSR has already wondered whether it will become the "Whole Foods of fast food."

At Lyfe, the cookies are dairy-free; the beef comes from grass-fed, humanely raised cows; nothing weighs in at more than 600 calories; and there's no butter, cream, white sugar, white flour, high-fructose corn syrup, or trans fats. The concept was the brainchild of the former Gardein executive and investment banker Stephen Sidwell, who quickly enlisted Mike Roberts, the former global president of McDonald's, and Mike Donahue, McDonald's U.S.A.'s chief of corporate communications. These three teamed up with Art Smith, Oprah's former chef, and Tal Ronnen, who I believe to be among the most ambitious and talented vegan chefs in the country.

According to Roberts, Lyfe currently has more than 250 angel investors who "represent a group of people that are saying, 'We've been waiting for something like this.'" The Culver City operation opened earlier this year, and two more California locations are scheduled to open before the year is out. New York locations are being actively scouted, and a Chicago franchise is in the works.

When I visited the Culver City operation, shortly before its official opening, I sampled across the menu and came away impressed. There are four small, creative flatbread pizzas under $10; one is vegan, two are vegetarian, and one was done with chicken. I tasted terrific salads, like a beet-and-farro one ($9) that could easily pass for a starter at a good restaurant, and breakfast selections, like steel-cut oatmeal with yogurt and real maple syrup ($5) and a tofu wrap ($6.50), were actually delicious.

Lyfe, not unlike life, isn't cheap. The owners claim that an average check is "around $15" but one entree (roast salmon, bok choy, shiitake mushrooms, miso, etc.) costs exactly $15. An "ancient grain" bowl with Gardein "beef tips" costs $12, which seems too much. Still, the salmon is good and the bowl is delicious, as is a squash risotto made with farro that costs $9—or the price of a "chickin" sandwich at Veggie Grill or a couple of Tendercrisp sandwiches at Burger King.

How in the world, I asked Roberts and Donahue, can they expect to run

250 franchises serving that salmon dish or the risotto or their signature roasted Brussels sprouts, which they hope to make into the French fries of the 21st century? Donahue acknowledged that it was going to be a challenge, but nothing that technology couldn't solve. Lyfe will rely on digital order-taking, G.P.S. customer location—a coaster will tell your server where you're sitting—online ordering, and mobile apps. Programmable, state-of-the-art combination ovens store recipes, cook with moist or dry heat, and really do take the guesswork out of cooking. An order-tracking system tells cooks when to start preparing various parts of dishes and requires their input only at the end of each order. Almost all activity is tracked in real time, which helps the managers run things smoothly.

Lyfe isn't vegan, so much as protein-agnostic. You can get a Gardein burger or a grass-fed beef burger, "unfried" chicken or Gardein "chickin." You can also get wine (biodynamic), beer (organic), or a better-than-it-sounds banana-kale smoothie. However, I fear that Lyfe's ambition, and its diverse menu, will drive up equipment and labor costs, and that those costs are going to keep the chain from appealing to less-affluent Americans. You can get a lot done in a franchise system, but its main virtues are locating the most popular dishes, focusing on their preparation, and streamlining the process. My hope is that Lyfe will evolve, as all businesses do, by a process of trial and error, and be successful enough that they have a real impact on the way we think of fast food.

Veggie Grill, Lyfe Kitchen, Tender Greens, and others have solved the challenge of bringing formerly upscale, plant-based foods to more of a mass audience. But the industry seems to be focused on a niche group that you might call the health-aware sector of the population. (If you're reading this article, you're probably in it.) Whole Foods has proved that you can build a publicly traded business, with $16 billion in market capitalization, by appealing to this niche. But fast food is, at its core, a class issue. Many people rely on that Tendercrisp because they need to, and our country's fast-food problem won't be solved—regardless of innovation in vegan options or high-tech ovens—until the prices come down and this niche sector is no longer niche.

It was this idea that led me, a few years ago, to try to start a fast-food chain of my own, modeled after Chipotle. I wanted to focus on Mediterranean food, largely on plant-based options like falafel, hummus, chopped salad, grilled vegetables, and maybe a tagine or ratatouille. I wanted to prioritize sustainability, minimize meat, and eliminate soda, and I'd treat and pay workers fairly. But after chatting with a few fast-food veterans, I soon recognized just how quixotic my ideas seemed. Anyone with industry experience would want to add more meat, sell Coke, and take advantage of both workers and customers to maximize profits. I lost my stomach for the project before I even really began, but recent trends suggest that there may have been hope had I stuck to my guns. Soda consumption is down; meat consumption is down; sales of organic foods are up; more people are expressing concern about GMOs, additives, pesticides, and animal welfare. The lines out the door—first at Chipotle and now at Maoz, Chop't, Tender Greens, and Veggie Grill—don't lie. According to a report in *Advertising Age*, McDonald's no longer ranks in the top 10 favorite restaurants of Millennials, a group that comprises as many as 80 million people. Vegans looking for a quick fix after the orthodontist have plenty of choices.

Good Fast Food doesn't need to be vegan or even vegetarian; it just ought to be real, whole food. The best word to describe a wise contemporary diet is flexitarian, which is nothing more than intelligent omnivorism. There are probably millions of people who now eat this way, including me. This flexibility avoids junk and emphasizes plants, and Lyfe Kitchen, which offers both "chickin" and chicken—plus beans, vegetables, and grains in their whole forms (all for under 600 calories per dish)—comes closest to this ideal. But the menu offers too much, the service raises prices too high, and speed is going to be an issue. My advice would be to skip the service and the wine, make a limited menu with big flavors and a few treats, and keep it as cheap as you can. Of course, there are huge players who could do this almost instantaneously. But the best thing they seem able to come up with is the McWrap or the fresco menu.

In the meantime, I'm building the case that it's possible to use real ingredients to create relatively inexpensive, low-calorie, meat-free, protein-dense, inexpensive fast food. If anyone with the desire can produce this stuff in a home kitchen, then industry veterans financed by private equity firms should be able to produce it at scale in a fraction of the time and at a fraction of the price. You think people won't eat it? There's a lot of evidence that suggests otherwise.

APRIL 3, 2013

It's the Sugar, Folks

Sugar is indeed toxic. It may not be the only problem with the standard American diet, but it's fast becoming clear that it's the major one.

A study published in the journal *PLOS ONE* links increased consumption of sugar with increased rates of diabetes by examining the data on sugar availability and the rate of diabetes in 175 countries over the past decade. And after accounting for many other factors, the researchers found that increased sugar in a population's food supply was linked to higher diabetes rates independent of rates of obesity.

In other words, according to this study, it's not just obesity that can cause diabetes: sugar can cause it, too, irrespective of obesity. And obesity does not always lead to diabetes.

The study demonstrates this with the same level of confidence that linked cigarettes and lung cancer in the 1960s. As Rob Lustig, one of the study's authors and a pediatric endocrinologist at the University of California, San Francisco, said to me, "You could not enact a real-world study that would be more conclusive than this one."

The study controlled for poverty, urbanization, aging, obesity, and physical activity. It controlled for other foods and total calories. In short, it controlled for everything controllable, and it satisfied the longstanding "Bradford Hill" criteria for what's called medical inference of causation by linking dose (the more sugar that's available, the more occurrences of diabetes); duration (if sugar is available longer, the prevalence of diabetes increases); directionality (not only does diabetes increase with more sugar, it decreases with less sugar); and precedence (diabetics don't start consuming more sugar; people who consume more sugar are more likely to become diabetics).

The key point in the article is this: "Each 150 kilocalories/person/day increase in total calorie availability related to a 0.1 percent rise in diabetes prevalence (not significant), whereas a 150 kilocalories/person/day rise in sugar availability (one 12-ounce can of soft drink) was associated with a 1.1 percent rise in diabetes prevalence." Thus: for every 12 ounces of sugar-sweetened beverage introduced per person per day into a country's food system, the rate of diabetes goes up 1 percent. (The study found no significant difference in results between those countries that rely more heavily on high-fructose corn syrup and those that rely primarily on cane sugar.)

This is as good (or bad) as it gets, the closest thing to causation and a smoking gun that we will see. (To prove "scientific" causality you'd have to completely control the diets of thousands of people for decades. It's as technically impossible as "proving" climate change or football-related head injuries or, for that matter, tobacco-caused cancers.) And just as tobacco companies fought, ignored, lied, and obfuscated in the '60s (and, indeed, through the '90s), the pushers of sugar will do the same now.

But as Lustig says, "This study is proof enough that sugar is toxic. Now it's time to do something about it."

The next steps are obvious, logical, clear, and up to the Food and Drug Administration. To fulfill its mission, the agency must respond to this information by re-evaluating the toxicity of sugar, arriving at a daily value—how much added sugar is safe?—and ideally removing fructose (the "sweet" molecule in sugar that causes the damage) from the "generally recognized as safe" list, because that's what gives the industry license to contaminate our food supply.

On another front, two weeks ago a coalition of scientists and health advocates led by the Center for Science in the Public Interest petitioned the F.D.A. to both set safe limits for sugar consumption and acknowledge that added sugars, rather than lingering on the "safe" list, should be declared unsafe at the levels at which they're typically consumed. (The F.D.A. has not responded to the petition.)

Allow me to summarize a couple of things that the *PLOS ONE* study clarifies. Perhaps most important, as a number of scientists have been insisting in recent years, all calories are not created equal. By definition, all calories give off the same amount of energy when burned, but your body treats sugar calories differently, and that difference is damaging.

And as Lustig lucidly wrote in *Fat Chance*, his compelling 2012 book that looked at the causes of our diet-induced health crisis, it's become clear that obesity itself is not the cause of our dramatic upswing in chronic disease. Rather, it's metabolic syndrome, which can strike those of "normal" weight as well as those who are obese. Metabolic syndrome is a result of insulin resistance, which appears to be a direct result of consumption of added sugars. This explains why there's little argument from scientific quarters about the "obesity won't kill you" studies; technically, they're correct, because obesity is a marker for metabolic syndrome, not a cause.

The take-away: it isn't simply overeating that can make you sick; it's overeating sugar. We finally have the proof we need for a verdict: sugar is toxic.

FEBRUARY 27, 2013

Is Alzheimer's Type 3 Diabetes?

Just in case you need another reason to cut back on junk food, it now turns out that Alzheimer's could well be a form of diet-induced diabetes. That's the bad news. The good news is that laying off soda, doughnuts, processed meats, and fries could allow you to keep your mind intact until your body fails you.

We used to think there were two types of diabetes: the type you're born with (Type 1) and the type you "get." That's called Type 2, and was called "adult onset" until it started ravaging kids. Type 2 is brought about by a combination of factors, including overeating, American-style.

The idea that Alzheimer's might be Type 3 diabetes has been around since 2005, but the connection between poor diet and Alzheimer's is becoming more convincing, as summarized in a cover story in *New Scientist* entitled "Food for Thought: What You Eat May Be Killing Your Brain." (The graphic—a chocolate brain with a huge piece missing—is creepy. But for the record: chocolate is not the enemy.)

The studies are increasingly persuasive, and unsurprising when you understand the role of insulin in the body. So, a brief lesson.

We all need insulin: in non-diabetics, it's released to help cells take in the blood sugar (glucose) they need for energy. But the cells can hold only so much; excess sugar is first stored as glycogen, and—when there's enough of that—as fat. (Blood sugar doesn't come only from sugar, but from carbohydrates of all kinds; easily digested carbohydrates flood the bloodstream with sugar.) Insulin not only keeps the blood vessels that supply the brain healthy, it also encourages the brain's neurons to absorb glucose, and allows those neurons to change and become stronger. Low insulin levels in the brain mean reduced brain function.

Type 1 diabetes, in which the immune system destroys insulin-producing cells in the pancreas, accounts for about 10 percent of all cases. Type 2 diabetes is chronic or environmental, and it's especially prevalent in populations that overconsume hyperprocessed foods, like ours. It's tragically, increasingly common—about a third of Americans have diabetes or pre-diabetes—and treatable but incurable. It causes your cells to fail to retrieve glucose from the blood, either because your pancreas isn't producing enough insulin or the body's cells ignore that insulin. (That's "insulin resistance"; stand by.)

Put as simply as possible (in case your eyes glaze over as quickly as mine when it comes to high school biology), insulin "calls" your cells, asking them to take glucose from the bloodstream: "Yoo-hoo. Pick this stuff up!"

When the insulin calls altogether too often—as it does when you drink sugar-sweetened beverages and repeatedly eat junk food—the cells are overwhelmed, and say, "Leave me alone." They become resistant. This makes the insulin even more insistent and, to make matters worse, all those elevated insulin levels are bad for your blood vessels.

Diabetes causes complications too numerous to mention, but they include heart disease, which remains our No. 1 killer. And when the cells in your brain become insulin-resistant, you start to lose memory and become disoriented. You even might lose aspects of your personality.

In short, it appears, you develop Alzheimer's.

A neuropathologist named Alois Alzheimer noticed, over a century ago, that an odd form of protein was taking the place of normal brain cells. How those beta amyloid plaques (as they're called) get there has been a mystery. What's becoming clear, however, is that a lack of insulin—or insulin resistance—not only impairs cognition but seems to be implicated in the formation of those plaques.

Suzanne de la Monte, a neuropathologist at Brown University, has been working on these phenomena in humans and rats. When she blocked the path of insulin to rats' brains, their neurons deteriorated, they became physically disoriented, and their brains showed all the signs of Alzheimer's. The fact that Alzheimer's can be associated with low levels of insulin in the brain is the reason why increasing numbers of researchers have taken to calling it Type 3 diabetes, or diabetes of the brain. Let's connect the dots: We know that the American diet is a fast track not only to obesity but to Type 2 diabetes and other preventable, non-communicable diseases, which now account for more deaths than infectious ones.

We also already know that people with diabetes are at least twice as likely to get Alzheimer's, and that obesity alone increases the risk of impaired brain function.

What's new is the thought that while diabetes doesn't "cause" Alzheimer's, they have the same root: an overconsumption of those "foods" that mess with insulin's many roles. (Genetics have an effect on susceptibility, as they appear to with all environmental diseases.) "Sugar is clearly implicated," says Dr. de la Monte, "but there could be other factors as well, including nitrates in food."

If the rate of Alzheimer's rises in lockstep with Type 2 diabetes, which has nearly tripled in the United States in the last 40 years, we will shortly see a devastatingly high percentage of our population with not only failing bodies but brains. Even for the lucky ones this is terrible news, because 5.4 million Americans (nearly 2 percent, for those keeping score at home) have the disease, the care for which—along with other dementias—will cost around $200 billion this year.

Gee. That's more than the $150 billion we've been saying we spend annually on obesity-related illnesses. So the financial cost of the obesity pandemic just more than doubled. More than 115 million new cases of Alzheimer's are projected around the world in the next 40 years, and the cost is expected to rise to more than a trillion of today's dollars. (Why bother to count? $350 billion is bad enough.)

The link between diet and dementia negates our notion of Alzheimer's as a condition that befalls us by chance. Adopting a sane diet, a diet contrary to the standard American diet (which I like to refer to as SAD), would appear to give you a far better shot at avoiding diabetes in all of its forms, along with its dreaded complications. There are, as usual, arguments to be made for enlisting government help in that struggle, but for now, put down that soda!

SEPTEMBER 25, 2012

Cereal? Cookies?
Oh, What's the Diff?

We all know the importance of real food in the morning: kids who eat high-sugar breakfasts have a harder time in school, and a growing body of research suggests that foods sweetened with sugar or high-fructose corn syrup can be as addictive as nicotine or cocaine. It's clear, too, that for most of us the eating patterns we develop as children hang around forever.

Every parent of a child born in the United States since 1950 also knows the difficulty of getting that kid to eat a breakfast of real food. This is not a "natural" inclination—no one is born craving Froot Loops or Count Chocula—but one resulting from a bombardment of marketing.

So for more than half a century well-intentioned parents have been torn between their desperation to get their kids to eat something, anything, and the knowledge that most packaged breakfast cereals are little better than cookies.

It turns out that from at least the perspective of sugar content, many are worse, as a document from the Environmental Working Group shows. There are at least 44 cereals that contain more sugar in a cup than three Chips Ahoy cookies. A cup of the most sugary cereal, Kellogg's Honey Smacks—they were called Sugar Smacks when I was a kid, but "Honey" is so much healthier-sounding, don't you think?—contains more sugar than a Hostess Twinkie.

So what else is new?

Not, certainly, the unchecked power held by junk food companies that brought us dessert disguised as breakfast in the first place; that's as old as the eight-track. Back in the '70s, consumer protection groups, prompted by increasing rates of childhood obesity, petitioned the government to regulate food marketing to kids. In 1978 the Federal Trade Commission (F.T.C.) issued proposed restrictions, but a few years and a few million dollars of food and advertising industry lobbying took care of those. By 1980 Congress had essentially stripped the F.T.C. of its authority to regulate marketing to kids.

Thirty years later, childhood obesity rates have tripled, PepsiCo is using horror computer games to sell kids Doritos, and the F.T.C. and Big Food are once again duking it out. Except it's a mismatch: Big Food is the heavyweight champ and the F.T.C. is an outgunned welterweight.

Earlier this year, a federal interagency working group (including the F.T.C.) submitted a draft of its recommended standards for marketing food and beverages to kids. The proposal effectively requests that manufacturers stop pushing junk to kids, at least that junk containing more than 15 percent saturated fat, 210 milligrams of sodium, or 13 grams of added sugar—about a tablespoon—per "serving." (Since the "serving sizes" used for calculations are usually unrealistically small, one tablespoon is in reality two.)

The proposed guidelines were completely voluntary, and while it seems unlikely that junk food companies ever intended to comply, they nevertheless pushed back hard against what they absurdly called job-killing regulation. At hearings held in October before the House Commerce and Health committees, they railed against the guidelines, and a recent report found that the food and advertising companies actively opposing the guidelines have spent more than $37 million on lobbying this year. (This number includes other lobbying efforts, but in any case, that's some serious clout.)

The same report found that Jo Ann Emerson, Republican of Missouri, the congresswoman who inserted language into an appropriations bill that would prohibit the F.T.C. from submitting a final draft of the guidelines before completing a full cost-benefit analysis, counts among her campaign donors PACs for PepsiCo, the American Beverage Association, and the National Restaurant Association—all of which have actively lobbied against the guidelines, of course. No conflict of interest there, and nothing surprising either.

Nor is it news that this lobbying is working. The F.T.C. is backing off some parts of its original guidelines, including constricting the target range from age 2 to 17 to age 2 to 11. (No doubt because 14-year-olds are mature enough to see through the marketing, right?) The agency is also no longer recommending that cartoon characters like Tony the Tiger or the Lucky Charms leprechaun be removed from products that fail to meet nutritional standards.

Let me remind you that the guidelines were voluntary in the first place.

How much more backing off can you do? We expect that the junk food industry is unwilling to agree to the F.T.C.'s increasingly lame voluntary standards. Why, after all, should they?

But here's what might be an actual surprise: The industry is even unable to follow the rules they themselves make. In response to the F.T.C. proposal, the Children's Food and Beverage Advertising Initiative (that's a junk food front group) released its own nutrition guidelines, which happen to allow almost 50 percent more sugar than the lax and voluntary number set by the F.T.C.

Only one-quarter of the 84 cereals reviewed by E.W.G. meet the F.T.C. voluntary guidelines. But that same number of cereals don't meet the lame guidelines that the industry set for itself. You read that right: Apple Jacks, the especially aggressively marketed Froot Loops, and 19 other cereals contain even more sugar than the industry's own guidelines recommend.

Regardless of the industry, self-regulation is a joke. What our kids are eating, on the other hand, is serious. And changing what they eat is going to require mandating—not requesting—the way that the junk food industry is allowed to manipulate them. The most important meal of the day is as good a place as any to start.

DECEMBER 8, 2011

Farmers' Market Values

For most of us, there's no better place to buy fruits and vegetables than at a farmers' market. Period. The talk about high prices isn't entirely unjustified, but it can be countered, and I'll get to that in a minute.

What's inarguable is that farmers' markets offer food of superior quality, help support smaller-scale farmers in an environment that's more and more difficult for anyone not doing industrial-scale agriculture, and increase the amount of local food available to shoppers. All of this despite still-inadequate recognition and lack of government support.

Then there's "know your farmer, know your food." When you buy directly from a farmer, you're pretty much guaranteed real freshness (we've all seen farmers' market produce last two or three times longer than supermarket produce). You're supporting a local business—even a neighbor! And you have the opportunity to ask, "How are you growing this food?" Every farmer I've spoken to says—not always in a thrilled tone—that the questions from shoppers never stop. But even if a vegetable isn't "certified organic," you can still begin to develop your own standards for what makes sense and what doesn't.

Farmers' markets are not just markets. They're educational systems that teach us how food is raised and why that matters.

"Producer-only" farmers' markets, as opposed to markets that sell food from anywhere, are really the ideal. The organizations that run these tend to be nonprofits, and often use volunteers to keep going. In many cases they are mission-driven: organizers want to make sure small farms remain viable and that we—nonfarmers—have access to good local food. At this stage of the game, there is no higher cause.

The quality of produce in producer-only markets—that is, places where people sell what they grow—is phenomenal, especially right now. If you're going to complain that tomatoes are $6 a pound in some markets (they are; they're also sometimes 99 cents), you might also note that usually these are real tomatoes, sometimes explosive in flavor, whereas the $4 per pound tomatoes I bought in the supermarket this week were grown in water and were less tasty than your average canned tomato. To some extent, you get what you pay for.

Then again, there are often bargains on incredibly high-quality produce for anyone who is willing to shop. Last week, at a recently opened market near Washington, D.C.'s convention center, I bought tiny lavender "fairy tale" egg-plants for less than $3 a pound. The Saturday before last, at New York's Union Square Greenmarket, I found perfectly ripe, real apricots for $5 a pound. (A chef strode up next to me and bought two cases; the farmer had only three total, which is why you want to go early.) That may sound expensive, but if you want a real apricot, this is the only way to get it.

At the 37-year-old market on 175th Street in Washington Heights, I found purslane—a salad green I've been foraging for 40 years, and that I adore—and bought a bunch as big as my head for $2. I found papalo (also called Bolivian coriander), a delicious, strong-tasting green I've bought every time I've seen it since I first tasted it in Mexico a few years ago.

And at the tiny farmers' market in Truro, on Cape Cod, now in its second year, I bought lobsters for 40 percent less than they cost in local stores, pork jowls for $2 a pound, and gorgeous half-yellow, half-green summer squash for a dollar each; they were worth it.

With more than 8,000 farmers' markets nationwide (representing something like 50,000 farmers, according to the Department of Agriculture), potentially millions of people are being affected by similar experiences. That's a great thing. And this week—National Farmers Market Week—a commemorative postage stamp is being introduced at a ceremony in Washington on Thursday. Present will be Bernadine Prince, co-executive director of FreshFarm Markets in Metro DC, which runs 13 producer-only markets, and president of the Farmers Market Coalition. Prince said to me, "Farmers' markets are an economic engine that keeps farmers going." Yes, that too.

That's good for everyone, but things could be better. It's clear to me—after visits to farmers in New York, New Jersey, Massachusetts, and California, to farmers' markets wherever I've traveled in the last few years, and recent conversations with Prince, Michael Hurwitz (director of New York's Greenmarket),

Francie Randolph (who runs Sustainable CAPE and founded the Truro market last year), and others—that a few key improvements could make it easier for farmers and markets to thrive.

Near the top of many lists is municipal support, largely in the form of space, water, electricity, and the like, and the reduction (or absence) of fees. "Each of our 13 markets requires a different negotiation and different set of fees," says Prince. "Some are a dollar a year and some are far more expensive." Since this money comes mostly from fees charged to farmers, the costs are usually passed on to consumers.

By increasing foot traffic, bringing shoppers into otherwise-ignored spaces, providing space for farmers to sell their goods at retail prices (80 percent of the farmers in New York's markets, says Hurwitz, could not survive on wholesale alone), these markets benefit everyone. Markets need infrastructure—either permanent space or, at least, water and electricity.

Farmers who come to market may be working 18-hour days, or even longer, depending on the length of their drive. On top of this, to handle retail sales they've got to process a variety of forms of payment in addition to cash, from SNAP (food stamps) to credit cards to tokens (you actually do not want to know how convoluted these payments get). When there's a unified, wireless form of payment, this will become less of a burden. That's in the works—Hurwitz estimates it'll be here no later than the end of the decade—but undoubtedly it could be hurried along.

At least a few hundred markets are taking advantage of programs like Wholesome Wave that double the value of food stamps at farmers' markets, and that number will soar when the Agriculture Department's Food Insecurity Nutrition Incentive program kicks in, contributing as much as $20 million to the cause. That's real progress, but more is needed.

In short, says the Southern Maine congresswoman Chellie Pingree, a staunch supporter of local food systems, "We've had some success in passing policies that support farmers' markets, but really the numbers are pretty small compared to the huge support that flows to big commodity crops. Policy makers are slowly catching up with the public on the benefits of supporting local agriculture, but we have a long way to go before the playing field is really leveled."

Truth.

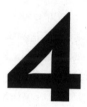

The Truth About Diet(s)

The standard American diet (or SAD, as many have come to call it) is a model for how not to eat. We consume far too many animal products (more than 600 pounds per person per year), sugary beverages and sweets (about a fifth of our daily calories come from those), and hyperprocessed junk food; meanwhile, the unprocessed fruits and vegetables that should be dominating our diets scarcely play a supporting role.

There's no lack of persuasive (and often deep-pocketed) corporations telling us what to eat, from the titans of the fast- and junk food industry peddling the myth that all calories are created equal, to gurus of fad diets that promote quick fixes over long-term health. The popular science confounds more than it clarifies, glorifying certain foods one year and demonizing them the next. In short, it's a minefield out there.

Adopting and maintaining a sane diet isn't easy, but it's more than doable. In this chapter, my thoughts on how (and how not) to eat.

(Only) Two Rules
for a Good Diet

SAN FRANCISCO—To a large extent, you can fix the food system in your world today. Three entities are involved in creating our food choices: business (everything from farmers to PepsiCo), government (elected and appointed officials and their respective organizations), and the one with the greatest leverage, the one that you control: you.

We shouldn't discount small farms and businesses, nor should we ignore relatively minor officials like the mayor of El Monte, Calif., who tried (and failed) to establish a soda tax to benefit public health. We do not always know where real change will come from, and certainly smaller operations may be more innovative and show us the way.

But for the most part we know where real change doesn't come from: Big Food, the corporations that supply most of the food and stuff masquerading as food that's sold in supermarkets, as fast food, and in casual dining chains; and government, especially the federal government, which is beholden to and entranced by big business. Nothing new here.

There often seem to be more happy exceptions in industry than in government. If you look at the relatively new companies that have blazed a path for the food industry, you see, among others, Whole Foods and Chipotle. One demonstrated that supermarkets could sell better ingredients; the other opened the door to non-junkie fast food.

Neither is above criticism, and it's possible both will be surpassed within a few years by newcomers with fresher and better ways of doing things. Still, it's comforting to know that at least somewhere in the corners of this food system, market competition is giving opportunities to clever and even well-intentioned people to figure out how to make real money by actually providing the public with better food.

I'm especially impressed with the way Whole Foods is innovating in the arena of labeling, gradually extending its own internal labeling system from fish to meats and now to fruits and vegetables. (As I said, though, they're hardly above criticism.) Marketing is of course part of it, but shoppers who want to talk back to the supply chain by knowing where their food comes from don't otherwise have a way to do that. If Whole Foods gives them what they want, then despite the "Whole Paycheck" nickname (and there's some evidence that Whole Foods is starting to compete on price as well), those who can get there and afford it will favor it. This is progress, doing well by doing at least some good, and that can't be said about most corporations involved in food. See, for example, the too-little-too-late attempt at transparency by McDonald's.

We can't rely on even well-intentioned souls in industry, but given the ball-dropping entity that is supposed to be vigilant regarding our health and welfare—the federal government—we have little choice. The legislative branch isn't worth discussing, and leadership from the executive branch has been disappointing. Two issues could have been improved definitively in the last six years—the marketing of junk to kids and the existence of antibiotics in our food supply—and President Obama has accomplished little in either case. However stymied he may have been, we are looking at a landscape that hasn't changed much, the exception being the improved but still hotly contested school food programs supported by the Healthy, Hunger-Free Kids Act.

Even worse are the Environmental Protection Agency, the Department of Agriculture, and the Food and Drug Administration, the last of which refuses to ban the routine use of antibiotics in animal production despite knowing that a ban is possible and desirable. It's also dawdling on mandating an improved nutrition label on packaged food, probably because of industry taking "interest."

We shouldn't need to rely on Whole Foods for good labeling. Yet every day I'm asked, "How do I know that what I'm buying is O.K.?" It seems the better educated and more concerned people are about this, the more confused they are. Drill deep enough and the list to worry about becomes overwhelming: organics, genetically modified organisms, carbon footprint, packaging, fair trade, waste, labor, animal welfare, and for all I know the quality of the water that's being used to wash your organic greens.

I get this. I'm a worrier, too, though I tend to expend my neurotic energy on different topics. The overall environment means that you're pretty much on your own if you try to eat healthfully in spite of the system, and you must take up that battle through a dozen or more decisions each day. But there are two big decisions that can put you on the right path and help you largely steer clear of antibiotics, excess sugar, unwanted chemicals, animal cruelty, and more.

Here, then, is your two-step guide for an unassailably powerful personal food policy.

> 1. Stop eating junk and hyperprocessed food. This eliminates probably 80 percent of the stuff that is being sold as "food."

> 2. Eat more plants than you did yesterday, or last year.

If you add "Cook your own food" to this list, it's even more powerful, but these two steps alone allow you to reduce the amount of antibiotics you're consuming; pretty much eliminate GMOs from your diet; lighten your carbon footprint; reduce your chances of becoming ill as a result of your diet; save money; cut way back on sugar, other junk, and unnecessary and potentially harmful nonfood additives; and so on.

All without relying on corporate benevolence or the government getting things right. The power lies with you.

OCTOBER 21, 2014

What Causes Weight Gain

If I ask you what constitutes "bad" eating, the kind that leads to obesity and a variety of connected diseases, you're likely to answer, "Salt, fat, and sugar." This trilogy of evil has been drilled into us for decades, yet that's not an adequate answer.

We don't know everything about the dietary links to chronic disease, but the best-qualified people argue that real food is more likely to promote health and less likely to cause disease than hyperprocessed food. And we can further refine that message: Minimally processed plants should dominate our diets. (This isn't just me saying this; the Institute of Medicine and the Department of Agriculture agree.)

And yet we're in the middle of a public health emergency that isn't being taken seriously enough. We should make it a national priority to create two new programs, a research program to determine precisely what causes diet-related chronic illnesses (on top of the list is "Just how bad is sugar?"), and a program that will get this single, simple message across: Eat Real Food.

Real food solves the salt/fat/sugar problem. Yes, excess salt may cause or exacerbate high blood pressure, and lowering sodium intake in people with high blood pressure helps. But salt is only one of several risk factors in developing high blood pressure, and those who eat a diverse diet and few processed foods—which supply more than 80 percent of the sodium in typical American diets—need not worry about salt intake.

"Fat" is a loaded word and a complicated topic, and the jury is still out. Most naturally occurring fats are probably essential, but too much of some fats—and, again, it may be the industrially produced fats used in hyperprocessed foods—seems harmful. Eat real food and your fat intake will probably be fine.

"Sugar" has come to represent (or it should) the entire group of processed, nutritionally worthless caloric sweeteners, including table sugar, high-fructose corn syrup, and so-called healthy alternatives like agave syrup, brown rice syrup, reduced fruit juice, and a dozen others.

All appear to be damaging because they're added sugars, as opposed to naturally occurring ones, like those in actual fruit, which are not problematic. And although added fructose may be more harmful than the others, it could also be that those highly refined carbohydrates that our bodies rapidly break down to sugar—white bread, for example—are equally unhealthy. Again: These are hyperprocessed foods.

In sum: Sugar is not the enemy, or not the only enemy. The enemy is hyperprocessed food, including sugar.

In the United States—the world's most obese country—the most recent number for the annual cost of obesity is close to $200 billion. (Obesity-related costs are incalculable but could easily exceed $1 trillion annually. Wanna balance the budget? Eat real food.) The amount the National Institutes of Health expends for obesity-related research is less than $1 billion annually, and there is no single large, convincing study (and no small study will do) that proposes to solve the underlying causes of obesity. If the solution were as simple as "salt, fat, sugar" or the increasingly absurd-sounding "calories in, calories out," surely we'd have made some progress by now.

We know that eating real food is a general solution, but a large part of our dietary problems might stem from something as simple as the skyrocketing and almost unavoidable consumption of caloric sweeteners and/or hyperprocessed carbs, which are in 80 percent of our food products.

Or it could be those factors in tandem with others, like the degradation of our internal networks of bacteria, which in turn could be caused by the overuse of antibiotics or other environmental issues. Or it could be even more complex.

The point is we need to know for certain, because until we have an actual smoking gun, it's difficult to persuade lawmakers to enact needed policies. (Smoking gun studies are difficult in the diet world, but throwing up our hands in the face of complexity serves the interests of processed-food pushers.) Look no further than the example of tobacco.

Meanwhile, if we had to pick one target in the interim, caloric sweeteners are unquestionably it; they're well correlated with weight gain (and their reduction equally well correlated with weight loss), Type 2 diabetes, and many other problems. How to limit the intake of sugar? A soda tax is a start, proper labeling would be helpful, and—quite possibly most important, because it's going to take us a generation or two to get out of this mess—restrictions on marketing sweet "food" to children.

There's no reason to delay action on those kinds of moves. But let's get the science straight so that firm, convincing, sound, evenhanded recommendations can be made based on the best possible evidence. And meanwhile, let's also get the simple message straight: It's "Eat Real Food."

JUNE 10, 2014

Which Diet Works?

One of the challenges of arguing that hyperprocessed carbohydrates are largely responsible for the obesity pandemic ("epidemic" is no longer a strong enough word, say many experts) is the notion that "a calorie is a calorie."

Accept that, and you buy into the contention that consuming 100 calories' worth of sugar water (like Coke or Gatorade), white bread, or French fries is the same as eating 100 calories of broccoli or beans. And Big Food—which has little interest in selling broccoli or beans—would have you believe that if you expend enough energy to work off those 100 calories, it simply doesn't matter.

There's an increasing body of evidence, however, that calories from highly processed carbohydrates like white flour (and of course sugar) provide calories that the body treats differently, spiking both blood sugar and insulin and causing us to retain fat instead of burning it off.

In other words, all calories are not alike.

You might need a little background here: To differentiate "bad" carbs from "good," scientists use the term "glycemic index" (or "load") to express the effect of the carbs on blood sugar. High glycemic diets cause problems by dramatically increasing blood sugar and insulin after meals; low glycemic diets don't. Highly processed carbohydrates (even highly processed whole grains, like instant oatmeal and fluffy whole-grain breads) tend to make for higher glycemic diets; less processed grains, fruits, non-starchy vegetables, legumes, and nuts—along with fat and protein—make for a lower glycemic diet.

A study published in the *Journal of the American Medical Association* adds powerfully to the notion that low glycemic diets are the way forward. (Or, actually, backward, since the low glycemic diet is largely traditional.) The work took place at the New Balance Foundation Obesity Prevention Center of Boston Children's Hospital, and looked at people's ability to maintain weight loss, which is far more difficult than losing weight. (Few people maintain even a small portion of their weight loss after dieting.) To do this, the researchers—led by the center's associate director Cara Ebbeling and director David Ludwig—put three groups of people on diets to lose 10 to 15 percent of their body weight.

They then assigned each of the dieters, in random order, to follow four weeks each of three diets with the same number of calories. One was a standard low-fat diet: 60 percent carbohydrates—with an emphasis on fruits, vegetables, and whole grains (but not unprocessed ones)—20 percent from protein, and 20 percent from fat. This is the low-fat diet that has been reigning "wisdom" for the last 30 years or more.

Another was an ultra-low-carb diet (for convenience, we'll call this "Atkins"), of 10 percent of calories from carbs, 60 percent from fat, and 30 percent from protein. And the third was a low glycemic diet, with 40 percent carbs—minimally processed grains, fruit, vegetables, and legumes—40 percent fat, and 20 percent protein.

The results were impressive. Those on the "Atkins" diet burned 350 calories more per day—the equivalent of an hour of moderate exercise—than those on the standard low-fat diet. Those on the low glycemic diet burned 150 calories more, roughly equivalent to an hour of light exercise.

Three conclusions you can draw on the face of this: One is that the kind of calories you eat does matter. Two, as Ludwig concludes, is that "the low-fat diet that has been the primary approach for more than a generation is actually the worst for most outcomes, with the worst effects on insulin resistance, triglycerides, and HDL, or good cholesterol." And three, we should all be eating an "Atkins" diet.

But not so fast; the "Atkins" diet also had marked problems. It raised levels of CRP (c-reactive protein), which is a measure of chronic inflammation, and cortisol, a hormone that mediates stress. "Both of these," says Ludwig, "are tightly linked to long-term heart risk and mortality."

His conclusion, then? "The 'Atkins' diet gives you the biggest metabolic benefit initially, but there are long-term downsides, and in practice, people have trouble sticking to low-carb diets. Over the long term, the low glycemic diet appears to work the best, because you don't have to eliminate an entire class of nutrients, which our research suggests is not only hard from a psychological perspective but may be wrong from a biological perspective."

Almost every diet, from the radical no-carb-at-all notions to the tame (and sane) "Healthy Eating Plate" from Harvard, agrees on at least this notion: reduce, or even come close to eliminating, the amount of hyperprocessed carbohydrates in your diet, because, quite simply, they're bad for you. And if you look at statistics, at least a quarter of our calories come from added sugars (7 percent from beverages alone), white flour, white rice, white pasta . . . are you seeing a pattern here? (Oh, and white potatoes. And beer.)

So what's Ludwig's overall advice? "It's time to reacquaint ourselves with minimally processed carbs. If you take three servings of refined carbohydrates and substitute one of fruit, one of beans, and one of nuts, you could eliminate 50 percent of diet-related disease in the United States. These relatively modest changes can provide great benefit."

The message is pretty simple: unprocessed foods give you a better chance of idealizing your weight—and your health. Because all calories are not created equal.

JUNE 26, 2012

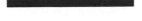

Will China Defeat Obesity?

S ay what you will about the Chinese, but they know how to make wholesale changes, and sometimes those changes are inarguably for the good.
As noted in an editorial in the *Lancet* last week, the life span of the average person in China in 1950 was 40 years; by 2011 it was around 76. (The average
life span in the United States in 2011 was 79.)

The causes of this near doubling of life span are no secret: China has developed public health programs that have reduced communicable diseases to
a manageable level. This is certainly good news. But it means that people are
now dying of noncommunicable diseases, or chronic diseases that are largely
preventable. These diseases, most common in wealthier nations, are caused not
by malnutrition in the classic sense but by overconsumption of disease-causing
foods as well as lack of exercise and environmental dangers.

Because things are moving so fast in China, and because that country can
learn from the example of the United States and others, perhaps it can pull off a
public health leapfrog and avoid the West's fate of a rapid and tragic increase in
obesity levels and the diseases with which they're associated.

And there's hope: The authors of the *Lancet* editorial wrote that Li Bin,
China's new minister of health and family planning, "has the political will, together with the support of international colleagues, to meet the urgent challenge" of these noncommunicable diseases and the problems they pose for
China's future.

In high-income countries, excess weight is the third-leading risk factor in
death. The importance of addressing this was brought home again last month
with the publication of a new study and editorial, also in the *Lancet*. The work

looked at 22 different cancers in Britain and their association with body mass index (B.M.I.), a simple but more effective measure of obesity than weight alone. The conclusions of the study, which involved a whopping 5.24 million people, were both notable and not entirely unexpected: When adjusted for factors like age and smoking, a higher B.M.I. was associated with a large increase in risk of cancers of the uterus, kidney, gallbladder, and liver, and smaller risk increases for at least six other types of cancer.

Most people are aware of the links among obesity, diabetes, and heart disease, but cancer is only occasionally discussed. And although that association is not news precisely, there are a couple of aspects of the new study that make it notable. The sheer size and carefulness of the study add credibility to the obesity-cancer link. And by showing that the more obese a person is, the greater the likelihood of his developing certain cancers, it's powerful.

The ways in which obesity makes an individual more prone to cancer are far from well understood. Finding those ways may lead to more successful treatment of cancer, and it's important and continuing work. But identifying what kind of policy might work to reduce obesity—regulations, taxes, subsidies for nonfattening foods, education about better diets, and so on—is, or should be, the primary work of public health officials, activists, and forward-thinking politicians.

With a staggering 70 percent of our adult population overweight or obese, the United States was until recently the world's leader in this unenviable race. Recently, Mexico (71.3 percent) took our place. (In China, the combined obesity-overweight rate is hovering at under 30 percent, still frightening.) Yet Mexico, which many Americans and Europeans haughtily consider primitive, was the first major nation in the world to institute significant soda and junk food taxes. That law went into effect early this year, and the results are already positive: Sales of soda are slipping.

In the 21st century, it is inevitable that nearly every citizen of the world has been and will continue to be affected by the scourge of junk food and liquid candy. Even though intelligent proposals abound, few countries have attempted to curb their marketing or sales. Without limits, the consumption of unhealthy foods will result in higher rates of obesity, and therefore an increase in associated diseases and premature deaths.

If we know how to diminish needless human suffering and mortality, why would we not? As Mexico has shown, it's the responsibility of government to protect its population from hyperprocessed food.

China has the potential to apply the lessons learned not only from its own positive experience dealing with communicable disease, but from the tragic mistakes made by so-called developed nations. It has a chance to turn the tide against disease-causing diets before it's too late. Sadly, we may need its example to wake up to our own problems.

SEPTEMBER 2, 2014

Butter Is Back

J ulia Child, goddess of fat, is beaming somewhere. Butter is back, and
when you're looking for a few chunks of pork for a stew, you can resume
searching for the best pieces—the ones with the most fat. Eventually,
your friends will stop glaring at you as if you're trying to kill them.

That the worm is turning became increasingly evident a couple of weeks
ago, when a meta-analysis published in the journal *Annals of Internal Medicine*
found that there's just no evidence to support the notion that saturated fat increases the risk of heart disease. (In fact, there's some evidence that a lack of
saturated fat may be damaging.) The researchers looked at 72 different studies
and, as usual, said more work—including more clinical studies—is needed. For
sure. But the days of skinless chicken breasts and tubs of I Can't Believe It's Not
Butter may finally be drawing to a close.

The tip of this iceberg has been visible for years, and we're finally beginning to see the base. Of course, no study is perfect and few are definitive. But
the real villains in our diet—sugar and ultra-processed foods—are becoming
increasingly apparent. You can go back to eating butter, if you haven't already.

This doesn't mean you abandon fruit for beef and cheese; you just abandon
fake food for real food, and in that category of real food you can include good
meat and dairy. I would argue, however, that you might not include most industrially produced animal products; stand by.

Since the 1970s almost everyone in this country has been subjected to a
barrage of propaganda about saturated fat. It was bad for you; it would kill you.
Never mind that much of the nonsaturated fat was in the form of trans fats,
now demonstrated to be harmful. Never mind that many polyunsaturated fats

are chemically extracted oils that may also, in the long run, be shown to be problematic.

Never mind, too, that the industry's idea of "low fat" became the emblematic SnackWell's and other highly processed "low-fat" carbs (a substitution that is probably the single most important factor in our overweight/obesity problem), as well as reduced fat and even fat-free dairy, on which it made billions of dollars. (How you could produce fat-free "sour cream" is something worth contemplating.)

But let's not cry over the chicharrones or even nicely buttered toast we passed up. And let's not think about the literally millions of people who are repelled by fat, not because it doesn't taste good (any chef will tell you that "fat is flavor") but because they have been brainwashed.

Rather, let's try once again to pause and think for a moment about how it makes sense for us to eat, and in whose interest it is for us to eat hyperprocessed junk. The most efficient summary might be to say "eat real food" and "avoid anything that didn't exist 100 years ago." You might consider a dried apricot (one ingredient) versus a Fruit Roll-Up (13 ingredients, numbers 2, 3, and 4 of which are sugar or forms of added sugar). Or you might reflect that real yogurt has two or three ingredients (milk plus bacteria, with some jam or honey if you like) and that the number in Breyers YoCrunch Cookies n' Cream Yogurt is unknowable (there are a few instances of "and/or") but certainly at least 18.

Many things have gone awry with the way we produce food. And it isn't just the existence of junk food but the transformation of ingredients we could once take for granted or thought of as "healthy." Indeed, meat, dairy, wheat, and corn have become foods that frequently contain antibiotics and largely untested chemicals, or are produced using hybrids or methods that have increased yield but may have produced unwanted results.

Although the whole "avoid saturated fat" thing came about largely because regulators were too timid to recommend that we "eat less meat," meat in itself isn't "bad"; it's about quantity and quality. So at this juncture it would be natural for a person who does not read volumes of material about agriculture, diet, and health to ask, "If saturated fat isn't bad for me, why should I eat less meat?"

The best current answer to that: It's possible to eat as much meat as we do only if it's grown in ways that are damaging. They're damaging to our health and the environment (not to mention the tortured animals) for a variety of reasons, including rampant antibiotic use; the devotion of more than a third of our global cropland to feeding animals; and the resulting degradation of the environment from that crop and its unimaginable overuse of chemicals, soil, and water.

Even if large quantities of industrially produced animal products were safe to eat, the environmental costs are demonstrable and huge. And so the argument "eat less meat but eat better meat" makes sense from every perspective. If you raise fewer animals, you can treat them more humanely and reduce their environmental impact. And we can enjoy the better butter, too.

MARCH 25, 2014

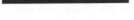

Can You Eat Too Little Salt?

TRAPANI PROVINCE, Sicily—On Sicily's west coast, there are two main crops: olives for oil and grapes for wine. There was once a third: salt.

Most high school students learn that salt was one of the motivating factors for the growth of the Roman empire, and that words for "salary" and "salad" come from the word for salt. Salt was a fundamental element of trade, because sodium and chlorine are both essential to life and the combination is among the best preservatives and flavoring agents there is. And until relatively recently, it wasn't easy to produce and ship, so overconsumption wasn't an issue.

Conditions for extracting salt from seawater are near-ideal here. There is unflooded flatland next to the sea, land that isn't great for farming; a long season that's both warm and dry; and lots of wind for both evaporation and power.

Early on, men figured out how to build a series of shallow rectangular ponds—called salt pans—and flood them with seawater during a spring high tide. As the water evaporated, it was moved into three or four subsequent basins until only a thick crust of salt remained. This was crushed, stored in covered piles, and sold. The development of windmills made the work easier and more efficient, so that by the middle of the last century annual production in the area reached nearly 200,000 tons, perhaps a 10th of a percent of the world's supply—not a big number but a thriving local industry.

Like most sea salt, the sea salt from Trapani has better flavor than land salt. I can't tell the difference in cooking, but the crystals from here—like those of other sea salts—are not only very salty but very flavorful. This isn't surprising, because sea salt is, after all, an extraction of the solids in seawater; most mined

salt is refined, and therefore pure sodium chloride, sometimes sold with iodide
or other additives.

None of this matters much now, except to the aficionado, the historian, and
the tourist. (On Sunday, I saw kids playing in piles of salt, as if it were snow. Yes:
It was weird.) The industrial mining of salt has all but ended the sea salt industry here and in many other places; there is a specialty market but it is more of a
relic than an integral part of the local economy.

When salt became cheap it became ubiquitous. No longer precious, it
began to appear in almost all foods, not just preserved ones. Perhaps it's easy
to overconsume in part because we have a natural taste for it, but of course it's
included—along with sugar—in processed foods, and in quantities that the majority of public health officials believe to be unhealthy, causing high blood pressure in formerly healthy individuals and exacerbating it in those with existing
high blood pressure. Eating less salt, generally speaking, causes blood pressure
to drop.

Enter Institutes of Medicine (or I.O.M., the medical branch of the National
Academy of Sciences), which has reported that as you go below 2,300 milligrams of sodium per day, the benefits are limited or nonexistent, and there may
be potential harm. But the report is far from conclusive (and a related paper in
the journal *Heart* has since been retracted), and the resulting kerfuffle, as far as
I can tell, is premature. (It could be that we discover that the whole controversy
is overblown, but the reigning wisdom, and the assertion of almost every public
health official internationally, is that too much salt is bad for you.)

In any case the report didn't mean that everyone can "go ahead and order
that side of fries," as the *Daily News* claimed. In fact, it changes nothing about
the general advice about salt and high blood pressure. It might mean, simply,
that you might not want to eliminate all the added sodium from your diet,
which would be nearly impossible anyway. (Milk contains sodium; spinach, too.
Nearly everything.)

In fact it's almost impossible not to get enough salt if you eat a decent diet
with a variety of foods, especially if you eat, for example, some bread or cheese
or pickles or canned tuna or . . . And even if you don't eat those things, unless
you exercise heavily in hot weather or get a flu that makes you vomit nonstop,
your chances of not getting enough salt are next to none. In short, you have
better things to worry about.

Of course you need sodium, but insufficient consumption is hardly a public
health threat. Even the I.O.M., which stoked the current version of this never-

ending controversy, found the evidence that it would be dangerous to aim for consumption below the recommended goal of 2,300 milligrams a day (for most people. For African-Americans and some other populations that appear to be more sensitive, it's lower) to be inconsistent, and called for more research. It may be true that there are no benefits in an ultra-low-salt diet, but almost no one is eating an ultra-low-salt diet. It's not quite like worrying about whether we get "enough" sugar, but it's nearly as ridiculous.

No doubt more research would be a good thing. But research is made difficult by the fact that 80 percent of the salt in the modern diet is in the processed food that you either eat at retail or in restaurants, not the food that you cook. Ten percent is naturally occurring; 10 percent is added at the table. The following chart from the Centers for Disease Control shows the big 10 suppliers of sodium in our diet and, though it's a bit opaque, one can gather that these are mostly if not entirely industry-produced foods.

The fact that most Americans eat the majority of their salt with little choice in the matter—and without knowing it—makes studies based on people's reports of their diets of questionable value. Many are consuming twice the daily recommendation, and many are consuming far more than that. The big, controlled studies that might really put this issue to rest are extremely difficult to execute, but without those studies, truly conclusive evidence is going to be impossible to come by, or nearly so.

Still: most people with high blood pressure respond well to a low-salt diet; and high blood pressure was not a problem in tribes scientists managed to find that still had diets containing no processed food. (That proves little, I know. If you want to argue that processed food is a bigger problem than salt, I'm with you.) It does seem that as sodium intake in a population decreases, so does blood pressure, so public health officials argue—not insensibly—that most Americans (probably 90 percent!) would be smart to try to eat less salt.

But how do you do that? By waiting for food manufacturers to figure out how to get unnatural foods to taste good with less salt in them? We've seen what happens when they try to cut fat: they add sugar. When and if they cut sodium, they'll do so by adding some weird ingredient or other (like potassium chloride, which has problems of its own), and 10 years down the road, or 50, it'll turn out that was worse for us than salt.

Here's the thing: Salt intake—like weight, and body mass index—is a convenient baseline for public policy people to talk about. If you focus on eating less salt—and, indeed, less sugar—you will inevitably eat less processed food, fast food, junk food (it's all the same thing). If you eat less processed food (etc.) you eat more real food. If you eat more real food, not only are you healthier, but you probably don't have to pay attention to how much salt you're eating.

MAY 28, 2013

TABLE 1. Ranked population proportions of sodium consumed, by selected food categories and age groups—*What We Eat in America* (*WWEIA*), National Health and Nutrition Examination Survey, United States, 2007–2008

RANK	FOOD CATEGORY	AGE GROUP (YRS)								
		≥2 %(SE)	2–19 %(SE)	2–5 %(SE)	6–11 %(SE)	12–19 %(SE)	≥20 %(SE)	20–50 %(SE)	51–70 %(SE)	≥71 %(SE)
1	Breads and rolls	7.4 (0.2)	6.9 (0.4)	6.5 (0.5)	7.8 (0.6)	6.5 (0.4)	7.5 (0.2)	7.2 (0.3)	7.8 (0.4)	9.6 (0.3)
2	Cold cuts/ cured meats	5.1 (0.3)	4.4 (0.4)	3.4 (0.5)	4.3 (0.4)	4.9 (0.7)	5.3 (0.3)	5.5 (0.5)	4.6 (0.2)	6.0 (0.5)
3	Pizza	4.9 (0.2)	7.3 (0.4)	4.8 (0.7)	7.2 (0.6)	8.2 (0.7)	4.1 (0.2)	5.0 (0.4)	3.0 (0.4)	1.7 (0.2)
4	Poultry	4.5 (0.2)	5.5 (0.4)	5.5 (0.4)	4.7 (0.4)	6.0 (0.6)	4.2 (0.3)	4.5 (0.3)	3.9 (0.3)	2.7 (0.3)
5	Soups	4.3 (0.3)	4.0 (0.2)	5.3 (0.9)	3.6 (0.4)	3.9 (0.4)	4.4 (0.4)	4.2 (0.4)	4.6 (0.7)	5.7 (0.7)
6	Sandwiches	4.0 (0.3)	4.4 (0.3)	3.5 (0.3)	3.9 (0.3)	5.0 (0.5)	3.9 (0.3)	4.5 (0.3)	3.2 (0.6)	3.7 (0.5)
7	Cheese	3.8 (0.2)	3.8 (0.3)	4.2 (0.4)	3.7 (0.3)	3.9 (0.4)	3.8 (0.2)	3.9 (0.2)	3.5 (0.2)	1.8 (0.3)
8	Pasta mixed dishes	3.3 (0.2)	3.8 (0.4)	4.0 (0.6)	4.0 (0.5)	3.7 (0.4)	3.1 (0.2)	3.4 (0.4)	2.4 (0.5)	2.9 (0.3)
9	Meat mixed dishes	3.2 (0.3)	2.1 (0.4)	—	2.2 (0.5)	1.9 (0.4)	3.6 (0.3)	3.5 (0.3)	3.6 (0.7)	4.2 (0.7)
10	Savory snacks	3.1 (0.2)	4.4 (0.3)	3.4 (0.2)	4.6 (0.4)	4.6 (0.6)	2.8 (0.2)	2.8 (0.2)	3.0 (0.4)	1.6 (0.2)
Mean daily sodium consumption (mg) (SE)		3,266 (40)	2,957 (53)	2,245 (54)	2,944 (72)	3,310 (70)	3,372 (48)	3,568 (58)	3,239 (73)	2,658 (77)
Unweighted no. of participants in sample		7,221	2,544	662	901	981	4,683	2,280	1,549	854

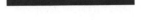

Got Milk? You Don't Need It

Drinking milk is as American as Mom and apple pie. Until not long ago, Americans were encouraged not only by the lobbying group called the American Dairy Association but by parents, doctors, and teachers to drink four 8-ounce glasses of milk, "nature's perfect food," every day. That's two pounds! We don't consume two pounds a day of anything else; even our per capita soda consumption is "only" a pound a day.

These days the Department of Agriculture's recommendation for dairy is a mere three cups daily—still 1½ pounds by weight—for every man, woman, and child over age 9. This in a country where as many as 50 million people are lactose intolerant, including 90 percent of all Asian-Americans and 75 percent of all African-Americans, Mexican-Americans, and Jews. The myplate.gov site helpfully suggests that those people drink lactose-free beverages. (To its credit, it now counts soy milk as "dairy.")

There's no mention of water, which is truly nature's perfect beverage; the site simply encourages us to switch to low-fat milk. But, says Neal Barnard, president of the Physicians Committee for Responsible Medicine, "Sugar—in the form of lactose—contributes about 55 percent of skim milk's calories, giving it ounce for ounce the same calorie load as soda."

O.K., dairy products contain nutrients, and for those who like them, a serving or two daily is probably fine. (Worth noting: they're far more easily digested as yogurt or cheese than as fluid milk.) But in addition to intolerance, there's a milk allergy—the second most common food allergy after peanuts, affecting an estimated 1.3 million children—that can be life-threatening.

Other conditions are not easily classified, and I have one of those. When

I was growing up, drinking milk at every meal, I had a chronic upset stomach. (Channeling my inner Woody Allen, I'll note that I was therefore treated as a neurotic, which, in fairness, I was anyway.) In adolescence, this became chronic heartburn, trendily known as GERD or acid reflux, and that led to a lifelong Tums habit (favorite flavor: wintergreen) and an adult dependence on Prevacid, a proton-pump inhibitor. Which, my gastroenterologist assured me, is benign. (Wrong.)

Fortunately my long-term general practitioner, Sidney M. Baker, author of *Detoxification and Healing*, insisted that I make every attempt to break the Prevacid addiction. Thus followed a seven-year period of trials of various "cures," including licorice pills, lemon juice, antibiotics, famotidine (Pepcid), and almost anything else that might give my poor, sore esophagus some relief. At some point, Dr. Baker suggested that despite my omnivorous diet I consider a "vacation" from various foods.

So, three months ago, I decided to give up dairy products as a test. Twenty-four hours later, my heartburn was gone. Never, it seems, to return. In fact, I can devour linguine puttanesca (with anchovies) and go to bed an hour later; fellow heartburn sufferers will be impressed. Perhaps equally impressive is that I mentioned this to a friend who had the same problem, tried the same approach, and had the same results. Presto! No dairy, no heartburn! (A third had no success. Hey, it's not a controlled double-blind experiment, but there is no downside to trying it.)

Conditions like mine are barely on the radar. Although treating heartburn is a business worth more than $10 billion a year, the solution may be as simple as laying off dairy. (Which, need I point out, is free.) What's clear is that the widespread existence of lactose intolerance, says Dr. Baker, is "a pretty good sign that we've evolved to drink human milk when we're babies but have no need for the milk of any animals. And no matter what you call a chronic dairy problem—milk allergy, milk intolerance, lactose intolerance—the action is the same: avoid all foods derived from milk for at least five days and see what happens."

Adds Dr. Barnard, "It's worth noting that milk and other dairy products are our biggest source of saturated fat, and there are very credible links between dairy consumption and both Type 1 diabetes and the most dangerous form of prostate cancer." Then, of course, there are our 9 million dairy cows, most of whom live tortured, miserable lives while making a significant contribution to greenhouse gases.

But what about the bucolic cow on the family farm? What about bone density and osteoporosis? What about Mom, and apple pie?

Mom: Don't know about yours, but mine's doing pretty well. Apple pie (best made with one crust, plenty of apples) will be fine.

But the bucolic cow and family farm barely exist: "Given the Kafkaesque federal milk marketing order system, it's impossible for anyone to make a living producing and selling milk," says Anne Mendelson, author of *Milk*. "The exceptions are the very largest dairy farms, factory operations with anything from 10,000 to 30,000 cows, which can exploit the system, and the few small farmers who can opt out of it and sell directly to an assured market, and who can afford the luxury of treating the animals decently."

Osteoporosis? You don't need milk, or large amounts of calcium, for bone integrity. In fact, the rate of fractures is highest in milk-drinking countries, and it turns out that the keys to bone strength are lifelong exercise and vitamin D, which you can get from sunshine. Most humans never tasted fresh milk from any source other than their mother for almost all of human history, and fresh cow's milk could not be routinely available to urbanites without industrial production. The federal government not only supports the milk industry by spending more money on dairy than any other item in the school lunch program, but by contributing free propaganda as well as subsidies amounting to well over $4 billion in the last 10 years.

There's nothing un-American about re-evaluating those commitments with an eye toward sensibility. Meanwhile, pass the water.

More on Milk

When I wrote about my experiences with giving up dairy, I heard from many hundreds of readers who attributed to dairy health problems as varied as heartburn, migraines, irritable bowel syndrome, colitis, eczema, acne, hives, asthma ("When I gave up dairy, my asthma went away completely"), gallbladder issues, body aches, ear infections, colic, "seasonal allergies," rhinitis, chronic sinus infections, and more. (One writer mentioned an absence of canker sores after cutting dairy; I realized I hadn't had a canker sore—which I've gotten an average of once a month my whole life—in four months. Something else to think about.)

Although lactose intolerance and its generalized digestive tract problems are well documented, and milk allergies are thought to affect perhaps 1 percent of the American population, the links between milk (or dairy) and such a broad range of ailments has not been well studied, at least by the medical establishment.

Yet if you speak with people who've had these kinds of reactive problems, it would appear that the medical establishment is among the last places you'd want to turn for advice. Nearly everyone who complained of heartburn, for example, later resolved by eliminating dairy, had a story of a doctor (usually a gastroenterologist) prescribing a proton-pump inhibitor, or P.P.I., a drug (among the most prescribed in the United States) that blocks the production of acid in the stomach.

But—like statins—P.P.I.s don't address underlying problems, nor are they "cures." They address only the symptom, not its cause, and they are only effective while the user takes them. Thus in the last few days I've read scores of stories like mine, some of which told of involuntary or incidental withdrawal of dairy from the diet—a trip to China (where milk remains less common), or a vacation with non-milk-drinking friends or family—when symptoms disappeared, followed by their return upon resumption of a "normal" diet.

Others abandoned dairy for animal cruelty reasons, or a move towards veganism, and found, as one reader wrote, "My chronic lifelong nasal congestion vanished within a week, never to return." Still others (I'm happy to report) read my piece and, like one writer, "immediately gave up dairy . . . and quit taking my medications. After nine days . . . I have had no heartburn, despite the fact that I have eaten many foods that would normally bring it on. . . . It feels like a miracle."

There is anger as well as surprise, because you'd think that with a grapevine's worth of anecdotal stories and at least some studies linking dairy to physical problems, few people began this kind of self-testing at the suggestion of their doctor—unless, that is, their doctor was in the "alternative" camp.

So I got mail saying things like, "When I think back to all the things I've missed because I had a migraine, it makes me a little angry that the solution for me was so simple." When a lifetime of suffering, medical visits, and prescription drugs can be resolved with a not especially challenging dietary change—one that, when it works, has rewards well worth the sacrifice—a certain amount of retroactive frustration seems justifiable.

I don't want to give the impression that the response was uniform. Though it was overwhelmingly in tune with my own experience, there are people who insist that the symptoms don't come from all milk but "American" milk (this doesn't happen in Europe, some say), or pasteurized milk (raw milk is the answer) or cow's milk ("goat's milk doesn't cause problems") or uncooked milk, or nonorganic milk, or only milk—that is, that yogurt and cheese don't cause the same kinds of problems. Others suggested that it's not milk but coffee that's the problem (and for at least one writer, that was undoubtedly the case), or that milk—as was thought when I was growing up, and my father drank it to ease his ulcer—was soothing rather than irritating.

All of this, of course, can be true for some and not true for others. (It would not surprise me a bit if it were eventually discovered that industrial production methods, which include giving dairy cows feed that they have trouble digesting, produce an inferior and somehow damaging form of dairy.) I do think that on the basis of what appears to be widespread experience anyone with chronic heartburn or any of the other ailments mentioned above would be missing an opportunity if he or she didn't give a nondairy diet a shot. As Erik Marcus, who publishes Vegan.com, wrote to me, "In talking to other vegans I rarely hear them say they feel much different after quitting meat or eggs, but you hear all sorts of stories like yours and mine once they quit dairy."

The stories here expose problems both with agriculture and with medicine. Once American agriculture became fixated on producing the most crops possible, regardless of the cost to land, water, air, animals, and people, one of the jobs of the Department of Agriculture became figuring out how to sell all that produce.

Thus selling and therefore consuming milk and other dairy—whether it's good for you as an individual or not—became an all-American task. (It's effective, too: we're on track to produce 91 million metric tons of fluid milk this year, less than 15 percent of it by small farms.)

But the job of an agriculture department should not be to sell whatever crops our farmers can grow most efficiently, it should be to encourage the growth of crops that will benefit the greatest number of Americans. Those crops are not corn and soy, grown largely to create hyperprocessed food or animal feed (and in turn animal products), but an increasing variety of plants that can be directly eaten by humans.

As for medicine: for many doctors drugs are the answer to almost every condition, a situation that suits Big Pharma just fine. More than $13 billion worth of P.P.I.s were sold in 2010, so if as few as 10 percent of those people were helped by a dietary change, the makers of Nexium, Prevacid, and Prilosec would be feeling the pain. Not the same kind of pain felt by the millions for whom dairy causes problems, however.

JULY 24, 2012

Dietary Advice for the Gluttony Season

Now that the gluttony season is upon us, you may be re-re-re-evaluating your diet; or perhaps you'll be stewing on it four weeks from today, making commitments to do better before summer.

We are confused. Many people have the gnawing feeling that "nothing" is fit, safe, wise, or ethical to eat, and the $61 billion diet industry encourages us to dwell on this uncertainty. We buy too much of the wrong stuff because it is affordable, satisfying, plentiful, and aggressively marketed. Then we seek the cure for what that toxic regimen causes. It's a dizzying merry-go-round.

There's no question that the safety thing is confounding, and it's not something individuals can do much about: You can avoid some chemicals by eating organic food, but that's not an option for everyone. Besides, even that doesn't address issues involving heavy metals or salmonella or god knows what else in our food supply. These are environmental problems, and one governmental responsibility on which everyone ought to agree is that environmental problems should be regulated until they're solved.

But nutrition advice need not confound; in fact, it's simple and has barely changed since you were a kid (it doesn't even matter when you were a kid). "Eat a variety of foods" almost does the trick, if the foods you're eating are real, which means food with one ingredient or maybe four or six. (Most real bread, for example, is water, flour, yeast, and salt, with the possible addition of olive oil or a seasoning or two, and the possible subtraction of yeast. Yeast conditioners and ingredients with five syllables have no place in real bread.)

I asked Marion Nestle, who is among the wisest and sanest people I know when it comes to nutrition, how she might sum up dietary advice, and after noting that not much has changed since the '50s, she said: "The basic principles—then and now—are variety (eat many different kinds of foods to get all needed nutrients), balance (don't eat too much of any one food category, especially meat, dairy, and junk foods), and moderation (balance calories). To these, we can add: Eat more fruits and vegetables."

Some of this requires judgment, but it's safe to say that the less junk food (especially sugar and the like) and the more fruits and veggies you eat, the better off you are. We needlessly complicate things when we think about "nutrients" rather than "foods," and we often take rigid, extreme positions.

It was health warnings about cholesterol and fat that set off the low-fat, high-processed-carb craze, which led pretty much directly to the current obesity crisis. Indeed, if the nutrition advice of the '70s and '80s had been "eat most things in moderation, and don't eat too much junk," many pounds would have remained ungained. Instead we were told to eat low-fat foods, and we downed SnackWell's as if they were health food. Voilà.

When food is deconstructed into "nutrients" and we start worrying about how much oat bran or how little saturated fat we eat, we play a losing game, one that gives the marketers of processed foods—a very high percentage of which is not food at all—the opportunity to sell high-oat-bran or low-saturated-fat products as "healthy," regardless of their other properties.

Thus one purpose of "marketing" is "confusing," trying to persuade us that we must know a lot to make intelligent food choices. But little research on individual nutrients is conclusive. All you need really worry about is whether what you're eating is actually food, and if you're eating too much of one type, or simply too much. Except, again, fruits, vegetables, and other minimally processed plants, of which you'd have a hard time eating too much.

Which brings us to the extremism thing. On one end of the spectrum is the typical American diet, which is extreme in its contribution to chronic disease, environmental degradation, animal cruelty, and, we might add, setting a bad example. So we flee to the other end and deify veganism, now in the news every time someone famous announces they've "gone" vegan. The latest is that Al Gore has joined Bill Clinton in animal-free land, though there are the inevitable reports that maybe Clinton cheats. (Not that there's anything wrong with that.) Gore, presumably, finally recognized that the typical American diet of something like 600 pounds of animal products a year is inconsistent with a progressive or even realistic view of slowing global warming. Or maybe he just wanted to lose some weight. Or both—he didn't respond when I emailed him.

There's never any press when people simply decide to eat less junk food or more plants or less meat, yet both anecdotal and sales evidence show that meat consumption is down significantly in the United States. And yet it's the simple advice—the eat less meat and junk, eat more plants—that's going to make the biggest difference, because not only will more doctors and other advice-givers preach it but more people will also be able to heed it. Not likely true of veganism.

Besides, there's no guarantee that eschewing animal products will give you a healthy diet; it'll just give you a diet without animal products. (Jelly Bellys, Coke, and fries are all vegan.) It's true that veganism is an ethical response to the world's food problems (feed less to animals, and more to people) and it's obviously the only response if you don't want to kill animals to eat them, ever.

But there is logic to integrating animals into the agricultural landscape (Simon Fairlie makes that argument very well), and there is nutritional logic to eating some animal products.

Where there's no logic is in maintaining the status quo. I have no beef (forgive me) with vegans; in fact anyone who argues for a greater proportion of real plants in the diet is arguing for part-time veganism. But you don't need to go to the opposite end of the spectrum to avoid the standard American diet; you just need to follow the advice you already know.

DECEMBER 3, 2013

When Diet Meets Delicious

The "How do I eat?" thing has become increasingly combative and confusing. Do you give up carbs, or fat, or both? Do you go vegan or paleo? No. You eat like a Greek, or like a Greek used to eat: a piece of fish with a lentil salad, some greens, and a glass of wine. It's not onerous. In fact, it's delicious.

The value of this kind of diet ("diet" in the original, Latin sense of the word "diaeta," a way of living) has once again been confirmed in a study from Spain involving thousands of participants and published in this week's *New England Journal of Medicine*. So compelling were the results that the research was halted early because it was believed that the control group was being unfairly deprived of its benefits.

Let's cut to the chase: The diet that seems so valuable is our old friend the "Mediterranean" diet (not that many Mediterraneans actually eat this way). It's as straightforward as it is un-American: low in red meat, low in sugar and hyper-processed carbs, low in junk. High in just about everything else—healthful fat (especially olive oil), vegetables, fruits, legumes, and what the people who designed the diet determined to be beneficial, or at least less-harmful, animal products; in this case fish, eggs, and low-fat dairy.

This is real food, delicious food, mostly easy-to-make food. You can eat this way without guilt and be happy and healthy. Unless you're committed to a diet big on junk and red meat, or you don't like to cook, there is little downside.

On Monday I spoke by phone with Dr. Walter Willett, chairman of the nutrition department at the Harvard School of Public Health, who has been studying the Mediterranean diet for as long as I've been writing about food. His take was simple: "We have so many types of evidence that this kind of eating works, but the weight of evidence is important, and this adds a big stone to that weight."

As encouraging as the study is, it's far from perfect, and it would be hyperbolic—ridiculous—to say that it represents The Answer.

For one thing, the control group was supposedly on a low-fat diet, but didn't necessarily stick to it; in fact, it wasn't a low-fat diet at all. And the study did not show reversal of heart disease, as was widely reported; as far as I can tell, it basically showed a decrease in the rate of some cardiovascular diseases in people at risk as compared with people at risk who ate the typically lousy contemporary diet.

In short, as Dr. Dean Ornish said to me, "It's clearly better than a horrible diet, which is what most people eat." Dr. Ornish, who has devised a low-fat diet that has been demonstrated to reverse heart disease, said that "the most responsible conclusion from this study would be, 'We found a significant reduction in stroke in those consuming a Mediterranean diet high in omega-3 fatty acids, when compared to those who were not making significant changes in their diet.'"

Exactly. And that's good news, because it might encourage some of the majority of people who are not making significant changes in their diet. Most Americans eat so badly that even a modest change in the direction of this diet is likely to be of benefit. That was the revelation of the Mediterranean style of eating when it came to public notice a generation ago. (Next year is the 20th anniversary of the publication of Nancy Harmon Jenkins's *Mediterranean Diet Cookbook*.)

Since we're being all Med, I could say *nihil novi sub sole*—there's nothing new under the sun—but it's not exactly true. What's new is all the junk that has been injected into our foods and our diet since the end of World War II. What's not new is that eating real food is good for you.

You could say that the Mediterranean diet prohibits nothing that was recognized as food by your great-grandmother. Whole, minimally processed foods of almost any type can be included in a sound diet. Period.

Current research does not give us the kind of detail many of us crave. It may well be that the reason red meat appears to be "bad" for us lies in the way cattle are raised. It may well be that the reason wine appears to be "good" for us is that it's usually consumed as part of a leisurely meal with family or friends. My guess is that wild fish—which is in general endangered and cannot in good conscience be eaten as often as I, for one, would like to—is far more beneficial than farm-raised fish, which has mostly understated environmental issues.

But we don't need to resolve these issues to understand that eating real food—most often cooked by yourself, because getting real food in all but the best restaurants is a great challenge—is going to help you avoid chronic disease.

This probably means you should think about salads or rice and beans for lunch, because unless you're at home or your workplace has a super-duper cafeteria or you have loads of money and work next door to, I don't know, the Four Seasons, you're not going to have many better options. It probably means that breakfast should be oatmeal or fruit salad—or eggs, which were unrestricted in this study—because you're probably not going to whip up a Japanese breakfast. Snacks should be nuts or fruit or more vegetables or beans.

And it probably means you should take control over dinner. So you're looking at a vegetable dish or two, some legumes, and a piece of fish, all cooked in or dressed with olive oil, and maybe a little bit of bread (preferably whole grain).

For dessert, fruit, or at least a dessert based on fruit or nuts or both. (The researchers had their subjects steer clear of what they called "industrial desserts," and one might just as well take that a step further and say "steer clear of industrial food.") Good chocolate, by the way, appears to be just fine.

As does wine: The study's participants were allowed seven glasses a week. Though red wine has a substance called resveratrol that seems to protect against cardiovascular disease, I have a hard time believing you must drink wine to be healthy. (I have an equally hard time limiting myself to a glass a day.)

I started a similar regimen to the one just described a few years ago, and by every measure my health improved.

You could justifiably ask, "How many times do we need to hear what has long been intuitively obvious: eat more fruit and vegetables and less junk and red meat?" But most people don't, which—unless we begin to mandate dietary regulation—makes this Spanish study all the more powerful.

Consider this the bottom line: eating well is not deprivational, but delicious. It's difficult to make generalizations about the American diet of a century ago, but we do know that it didn't include junk food because junk food didn't exist, and it didn't include a lot of sugar because there wasn't that much around.

So start with what we imagine that diet to have been, and adjust it so that it includes more legumes, less red meat and dairy, and more olive oil and more fish.

This is hardly a sacrifice: think about a frittata, a pasta dish with more vegetables, simply prepared fish and a reliance on legumes. The reasonable diet can include rib-eye, too, and even bad cheeseburgers, but the point is that those are not staples but treats, like ice cream and cheesecake and Reuben sandwiches. It's kind of as simple as that.

Should you eat beans two times a week or two times a day? Should you drink wine even if you don't like it? Feh. I would just envision a typical mezze plate and you will probably see what foods should dominate the assortment that makes up your daily diet: very little meat and dairy; a great deal of legumes and vegetables; perhaps a bit of fish; bread; and not much else. Certainly no cheeseburgers or Lean Cuisine.

Healthful food is delicious food, traditional food, real food. There is nothing new here. Eat real food, watch it on the animal products, and—even if you're a few pounds overweight—you'll improve the chances of your living a healthy life into what might actually be your golden years.

FEBRUARY 26, 2013

Finding Your Comfort Food

"What," people ask me, "do you cook when you're not working?" The answer is pretty consistent: "pasta and fish and a vegetable, or pasta and salad and a vegetable, or salad and fish and a vegetable, or pasta and salad and fish and a vegetable." There are exceptions, of course, but there's a comfort level here and it's been this way for a long time, through different kitchens and domestic arrangements.

Here's the thing: In my professional life of finding, replicating, sometimes even "creating" recipes, my palate is up for anything. But when the work hat comes off, I fall into old and completely beloved habits.

The pasta-salad-fish-veg thing began in the '80s, when I had my first real gardens. In summer and fall, I would make a daily bastardized ratatouille and finish it by putting a piece of fish on top, then steaming that. Sometimes there was pasta underneath. Usually there was a salad. Occasionally there was bread, though now it seems superfluous. That set the pattern.

And I come by the pattern, if not the ingredients, quite honestly. My mother's comfort zone wasn't dissimilar while my sister and I were growing up in New York City in the 1950s and '60s. We usually started with a salad doused with Wish-Bone, though sometimes that was preceded by a slice of melon (often ripe, oddly enough; she has a knack for determining that), a half grapefruit on which sugar was tolerated, or canned fruit packed in sugar syrup. This was followed, almost always, by a piece of broiled meat (or chicken or, very, very rarely, fish), potatoes (most often mashed, though my mother made superior French fries), and a canned vegetable like green peas or (even worse) green beans.

The quality of the ingredients was occasionally better, but sometimes worse. Relying on memory is tricky, of course, but when I grew up they were still raising pigs in Secaucus; potatoes came from Long Island, onions from the "black dirt" area of upstate New York. There were real bakeries—the kind that are making a comeback—and stores specializing in fruits and vegetables, so in the summer the tomatoes and corn came from Jersey farms.

That said, the lettuce was almost always iceberg. Romaine was exotic and kale and arugula were unknown. Ten months of the year the tomatoes were packed in cellophane, orange, and nearly as hard as apples. Most root vegetables were perhaps too reminiscent of our ancestors' presumed reliance on turnips; all I know is we didn't eat them. (Now I adore them.)

Really, it wasn't all that bad; we had fewer choices—not necessarily a negative—and we knew much less. But although olive oil was sold in four-ounce bottles (I swear!), the hegemony of Big Food was in its infancy; the first time I saw a McDonald's was in 1967, and that was in Pennsylvania—there were none in New York City—and there were no microwavable "meals." TV dinners were a monthly treat.

Our options now are infinite, but they're healthy only if we steer clear of the processed food aisles. (And you can buy canned fruit salad with no sugar!) Most cooks understand that making a vinaigrette is the work of a moment. Broiling a piece of fish or meat, steaming a vegetable, making a sauce for pasta—these are simple tasks.

Sure, I make adjustments. My pasta sometimes becomes rice (or rarely, if I'm to be honest, a more exotic grain like quinoa or farro) and the fish may be seasoned in a Japanese style: I might lightly salt-cure it, or simmer it in a mixture of soy and mirin and ginger. In this case the salad dressing might get a touch of sesame oil in it, or even a little soy and ginger. My personal preferences don't matter much; I just have a comfort zone that's mine, and it's neither brilliant nor unusual.

I once asked the food scholar and writer Alan Davidson what he ate on lazy nights, and he said, "A tuna sandwich and a glass of milk." I have friends who seem to live on homemade pizza, others who top salad with a piece of chicken, those who frequently "dine" on (fresh-popped) popcorn and a big salad with herbs, oil, lemon, and salt. Some make stews on Sunday and eat them three times during the week. These are all modest but real options, especially when compared to fast food, takeout, and the like.

Everyone can find a cooking comfort zone. An updated version of the one established by my mother, circa 1954, is just fine, especially if you do without the sugary fruit salad and find a real vegetable to plug in for the peas. Meat and potatoes may not be the ideal dinner from a health or environmental perspective, but there's a big difference between cooking a broiled chop and mashed potatoes, and burgers and fries from a fast-food place. Finding a comfort zone in cooking—any comfort zone—is better than not cooking at all.

AUGUST 12, 2014

The Frankfurter Diaries

I ate two hot dogs the other day. And now I'm going to talk about my feelings about junk food.

The circumstances were these: an early meeting at the *Times*, "breakfast" of a banana (and lucky to have that), and a morning of activities controlled by others.

Then there was a drive to the Jersey Shore. Just shy of noon, we stopped at a Garden State Parkway rest area of the new style: a "choice" of bad fast-food joints rather than just one. I begged my colleagues for some time to have a bite to eat. (It was a day that would include no lunch break.)

The choices were: prewrapped sandwiches, like smoked turkey with provolone on "whole grain" bread (it wasn't); Burger King; Sbarro; TCBY; Quizno's; Starbucks; Nathan's. I was on the phone with a friend who largely shares my weaknesses and prejudices. I did not want a prewrapped sandwich, especially one that looked so dry and unappetizing. My first inclination was Burger King; he pronounced it "poison."

O.K., but what wasn't? Where was the real food? It didn't exist. I gravitated toward Nathan's. After all, I grew up going to Coney Island; my mother is from there. Nathan's may not ever have been the best hot dog in New York, but it was iconic. Probably most important, the hot dog is to me comfort food. And it had been a long time.

It's not even that I was disappointed, though I can't resist noting that the bun was cold and stale; this wasn't supposed to be a remarkable eating experience. It's that, predictably, I felt lousy afterward, as many people say they do after eating fast food.

Yet we continue to. Why do so many of us have trouble learning this lesson? Let's for the moment ignore the research that seems to indicate that the word "addiction" may not be too strong to describe our relationship with junk food. Let's also ignore the information in the books by David Kessler (*The End of Overeating*) and my *Times* colleague Michael Moss (*Salt Sugar Fat*) that describes the junk food producers' efforts to offer precisely the stuff we'll find physically and psychologically irresistible.

Instead, let's just examine our feelings: what are our ties to the food that we know is not only evidently bad for us in the long run but also makes us feel queasy almost immediately afterward and doesn't even taste good?

I know the answers for me, and I doubt they're unusual: it's about my "relationship" to Nathan's, to hamburgers, to pizza. It's about my childhood: at my parents' house the other day, one of my daughters found a picture of my sister and me at Coney Island, two happy kids who had probably just eaten at Nathan's and were about to have waffles and ice cream on the boardwalk. It wasn't unusual to come home from Coney Island sunburned and stomachache-y.

I rarely get sunburned anymore; I've learned that lesson. On the other hand, I don't really remember the sunburns. Or even the stomachaches.

I remember the hot dogs. Without trying to recreate anything, I can feel that I have an attachment to those foods of my childhood that I don't have even for the most luxurious foods I've learned to love since then. I feel—and David Kessler talks eloquently about this in his book—that every time I see a hot dog it's at least a minor struggle not to eat it. Walking through an airport, I think, must be like being on the 12-step program at a series of weddings with open bars.

You probably know what I'm talking about, though your own weaknesses might be different. Perhaps every human who's ever lived has felt the same way about the foods of their childhood; but very few people, relatively speaking, have grown up in the junk-food-laden America that was born in the second half of the 20th century and shows little sign of dying.

We can conquer some of these compulsions: my sweet tooth is pretty much gone, and I expect that's because I finally recognized that mass-produced sugary stuff just doesn't taste very good. I've made that same recognition with some of the modern adaptations of the food I grew up loving: the smell of most French fries, for example—cooked in whatever chemically extracted, malodorous oil they're relying on nowadays—turns my stomach.

Smelling the stuff before you eat it helps; thinking about the stuff before you eat it helps, too—but these steps may not be enough to counter your mind's memories, sensations, and yearnings.

I know that I need to forget the Platonic ideal of the hot dog that's lodged in my mind and concentrate on everything I know that's wrong with the current iteration of it: the chemicals, tortured animals, artificial flavors, unnamed ingredients, miserable execution.

But I also know that understanding and willpower aren't enough. I'm well aware that we're light-years away from a rest area without any junk food. It might be nice, however, if there were one offering a vegetable wrap or a big fat falafel sandwich with real vegetables. Would you not think there's a market for that?

APRIL 30, 2013

Bagels, Lox, and Me

On Sunday, I put on my running clothes, went out to the elevator, and pushed the button. In the time it took for my finger to travel from the wall back to my side, I'd decided that it was not a day for a run but for a trip to the market. I slipped a coat over everything and went to the store, where I bought bagels, lox, and cream cheese, along with some badly needed staples. I then came home and ate. (While, of course, reading the *Sunday Times*. Sigh. Sometimes it's tough to be a cliché.)

The run never happened, and that's unusual in my recent history; I was a near-paradigm of discipline this winter. And I'm pretty disciplined in my eating, too, at least during the day. But something happened Sunday, a combination, I suspect, of annoying little things that led to a short-lived mental breakdown. The cause isn't important; it's the response that most interests me.

Consciously, the combination of bagels, cream cheese, and lox doesn't even rate among my top 10 comfort foods. Getting a good bagel is more challenging than getting a good slice of pizza, on which don't get me started. I'm pretty much anti-farm-raised salmon in principle, and all the fancy names processors give it don't change that. Cream cheese is by definition bland; if I'd never eaten it before and you served it to me, I'd see no reason to waste my caloric allotment on it.

But none of that seems to affect my cravings. I wouldn't claim that turning to bagels and lox and the physical newspaper on a weary-feeling morning is a genetic disposition, but I do come by it honestly. In the 1950s, my father (who turns 91 today!) would send me out for "appetizing"—as these foods were called, for some reason buried in New York history—to "Sol's," on the corner of First Avenue and 19th Street. (I picked up the paper on the way home.) In the 1930s, his parents sent him out, to Southern Boulevard in the South Bronx.

(This is not strictly relevant but it is, I think, revealing: He was instructed to buy "a half of a quarter"—that is, an eighth of a pound. For a family of six, that translates to a third of an ounce per person. I will never forget the looks on my parents' faces when they first saw my older daughter grab an entire piece of lox—an ounce at least—and place it on a bagel.)

For 50 years, through my childhood, my adolescence, my adulthood, my kids' births and maturation, there were periodic Sunday mornings spent visiting my parents. And every time, there it was: the holy trinity.

Every family, every ethnic group, and every person can talk about their cravings. The comfort food of others rarely appeals to us; it's our own that matters. I know people who drool at the sight of a bowl of rice, who cannot possibly resist it and, almost needless to say, many people feel the same way about pasta. A Hmong I met a couple of years ago could eat quarts of a shredded cucumber soup that had sustained him as a child (to me its flavor was as subtle as cream cheese, and it didn't even have the benefit of fat). Last weekend I chatted with a third-generation Irishman whose wife is a vegetarian and does the cooking; he sneaks out once a week for meat, potatoes, and gravy. My younger daughter seeks comfort in white beans with garlic, oil, and greens, which I often made for her when she came home from school during a particularly poignant period of our lives.

Your environment teaches you what comfort food is. Until recently, before marketing penetrated every cranny of our being, family and friends had the biggest impact: the stuff that made them happy made you happy. You can self-train your way out if it, as many of us have, and save it for special occasions.

You don't need a study to understand that for most of us the foods we come to love as children are the foods that will cry out to us for the rest of our lives; we'll occasionally seek to regain those feelings. (Whatever their source. I feel the same way about mushy pillows, well-worn cotton T-shirts, a really beat-up couch, and the music from *Carousel*.)

But with food, it seems these preferences for traditional foods are fading. I don't think feeling sad about that makes me a reactionary; I think it's important not to rob children of these kinds of memories, and to encourage those cravings that are driven by genuine traditions. Even if your own comfort food isn't the world's "healthiest," it's almost certain to be real. It's almost certain to have a link to your family's tradition; it's even likely that it's a preference that began with your grandparents, or perhaps many generations ago.

I recognize that some of this loss is a result of the homogenization and general loss of ethnicity we sacrifice in becoming "American." I recognize that this is not a country rich with food traditions, though most of us crave some specific side dish—if not turkey—on the fourth Thursday of November.

But when childhood food preferences are formed around foodlike substances that were invented in the last 50 years by scientists and marketers looking to develop "food" that appeals to that same comfort-craving part of your brain—without any consideration of tradition or quality—that's a bad situation. If a marketer can make it so that you feel the same way about a bacon double cheeseburger as you do about the special beans-and-greens or roast chicken your grandmother made for you, and then he makes that double cheeseburger available to you almost everywhere you go, he's got you locked in forever. That's just not the same thing as bagels and lox.

APRIL 29, 2014

Why I'm Not a Vegan

When I am asked for my take on a positive direction for the American diet, the answer seems obvious. I've been semi-vegan for six years and in this column as well as my book *VB6* (for "Vegan Before 6 p.m."), I argue that this strategy, or one like it, can move us toward better health. (I eat mostly unprocessed plants before 6 p.m., and then whatever I want afterward. And, in answer to the most frequently asked question: Yes, I cheat.)

In the last 30 years, researchers have graduated from the notion that Americans should "eat less fat, especially saturated fat"—the catchphrase of '80s nutritionists, which led to "low-fat" foods (SnackWell's is a shining but hardly only example) and the biggest per capita weight gain in American history—to widespread agreement that we eat too few unprocessed plants and too much hyperprocessed food, especially food containing sugar and those carbohydrates that our bodies convert rapidly to sugar. There is also compelling evidence that we eat too many animal products (something like 600 pounds per person per year) and too much salt.

None of this is simple. For one thing, we still have much to learn about the composition of plants and the aspects of them that are good for us (as David Katz has said, "The active ingredient in broccoli is broccoli"), although it's becoming clear that they're beneficial not so much as a combination of nutrients but as the right package of nourishment, which we might as well call real food. In other words, you're better off eating a carrot than the beta-carotene that was once thought to be its most beneficial "ingredient." And for another, salt and sugar are necessary parts of a sound diet, but so much of each is added to processed food that we're getting way too much of both. It's likely that neither would be a concern if we were doing all of our cooking from scratch, but of course we are not.

Animal products have a special place in this discussion, because unlike hyperprocessed foods they have been a part of the diet of most humans since humans existed, and because their concentration of nutrients makes consuming at least some of them convenient and perhaps even smart.

There is, however, a limit to their benefit. Until recently, even "successful" agriculture failed to guarantee unlimited animal products to the masses, but industrial agriculture changed that, and, since (say) 1950, almost anyone in a developed country who could afford (say) a car could also afford to eat meat, dairy, and/or eggs as often as he liked.

Although the most convincing research indicates that red meat is the least healthy, it also appears that those who turn to what's called a "paleo" diet—one comprising primarily meat, fruits, and vegetables but not so much in the way of legumes or grains—may avoid some of the pitfalls of the standard American diet but still fall prey to others.

Besides, there are non-dietary reasons to eat fewer animal products. Even if their nutritional profile were unambivalently beneficial, they use too many resources: land, water, energy, and—not the least important—food that could nourish people. And livestock is a major (if not the leading) contributor to greenhouse gases, while the rampant and nearly unregulated use of antibiotics in that production is making those drugs less effective and encouraging the development of hardier disease-causing germs.

From every perspective, then, it seems we should be eating more plants and less of everything else. "So," a certain percentage of the people I spoke to this month asked, "why not go whole hog" (forgive me) "and advocate a strictly vegan diet?" Isn't being a part-time vegan, the more strident demand, like being a little bit pregnant?

To that last question, the answer is, "Obviously not." A vegan meal has no implications about what your next meal may be; you can be vegan for the better part of a day, or for a number of days of your life. Part-time veganism (which you might also call flexitarianism) is a strategy for integrating the reigning wisdom—eat more plants, less hyperprocessed stuff, fewer animal products—into lives that have, until now, been composed of too few of the first and too many of the second and third.

VB6 is just one such strategy; in my travels, I met people who were "vegan until the weekend" or vegan all but five days a month, or any number of other approaches to achieving the same goal. You might think of patterns of eating as falling on one point or another along a spectrum, and moving toward the plant-based end of that spectrum—as opposed to the end represented by Morgan Spurlock's "super-sized" diet—is almost always beneficial. It is about eating better, or well, not perfectly, and it must be said that "perfectly" has not yet been defined. (A vegan diet is no guarantee of a good diet, unless the only goal is to avoid killing animals. Sugar-sweetened beverages, French fries, and doughnuts can all be vegan.)

I can see three scenarios that might lead to universal, full-time veganism: An indisputable series of research results proving that consuming animal products is unquestionably "bad" for us; the emerging dominance of a morality that asserts that we have no right to "exploit" our fellow animals for our own benefit; or an environmental catastrophe that makes agriculture as we know it untenable. All seem unlikely.

This much is known, now: We produce most animal products in deplorable conditions, and some of our health and environmental problems can be traced both to dominant production methods and our overconsumption. But we like to eat them, and they're a pleasurable and even healthy part of many traditional diets and even sound agricultural practices.

So: reduce the rate at which we consume animal products, produce them better, and substitute plants for a large portion of them. We'll improve our health, animal welfare, and the state of the environment. Not a bad bargain.

MAY 21, 2013

5

The Broken Food Chain

The industrialization of American meat production and junk-ification of the standard American diet have together created a public health crisis of super-sized proportions. Factory farms routinely churn out food-borne illnesses and antibiotic-resistant bacteria, while a culture of unhealthy eating has produced what can only be described as a pandemic of preventable lifestyle diseases that not only kill at an alarming rate, but cost an absolute fortune to treat—some say as much as a trillion dollars a year.

Of course, it's not just consumers who are endangered by our food system, but workers as well. I'm talking about people who labor at every step of the food chain: farmworkers who may be quite literally enslaved, restaurant cooks sneezing on your food because they don't get paid sick leave, servers—what used to be called waiters and waitresses—denied their tips by crooked managers, and countless fast-food workers making far less than a living wage. Without justice for them—not to mention food service workers, supermarket clerks, shelf stockers, slaughterhouse workers, you get the idea—there is no such thing as fair and "healthy" food.

Dietary Seat Belts

Here's some good news: Seat belts save lives, a lot of them. So do vaccinations. The childhood obesity rate has declined (a little) in parts of the United States. That last thing is miraculous, because the policies for food, energy, climate change, and health care are, effectively, "let's help big producers make as much money as they can regardless of the consequences."

Except for just after the most visible tragedies, public health and welfare are barely part of the daily conversation. When New York is flooded, climate change dominates TV news—for a week. When innocents are slaughtered with weapons designed for combat, gun control is a critical topic—for a week. When 33 people die violent, painful deaths from eating cantaloupe, food safety is in the headlines—for a week. When nearly 70,000 people die a year, from mostly preventable diabetes, most media ignore it.

Forget the fiscal cliff: we've long since fallen off the public health cliff. We need consistent policies that benefit a majority of our citizens, even if it costs corporations money.

And guns are just the bloodiest public health menace to go virtually unregulated. Preventable, chronic disease—to a large extent brought about by diet—is now the biggest killer on the planet. Soda kills more people than guns—more people than car wrecks—only less dramatically. What we need is the equivalent of a dietary seat belt.

When we hear about extended life expectancy on a global scale (note that the country with the world's biggest economy—the U.S.—has the 51st highest life expectancy, just ahead of Taiwan and Chile, and roughly 20 places behind Jordan and Greece), we're hearing about the triumph of public health policies—

from municipal water treatment and delivery to sewer systems and immunizations. We're also hearing about health care that extends lives despite chronic disease, a triumph of expensive technology over thoughtful, less expensive planning.

And we're hearing about the failure of policy to address the leading public health challenge of the 21st century: not finding a "cure" for our leading killers—coronary artery and related disease, cancer, diabetes (which jumped from the world's 15th rated killer to its 9th in 20 years)—but taking easily defined action to prevent them.

The global burden of disease report found an impressive decrease in childhood mortality and deaths from malnutrition but also found a doubling of deaths from diabetes since 1990. Stroke and heart disease—not exclusively the result of obesity, but tied to it—are together responsible for a quarter of all deaths worldwide.

Malnutrition in the form of overeating is now a bigger problem than starvation, and both are preventable by sane policy measures that could make decent and real food available to all. Contrary to the hysterical preaching of techno-agriculturalists, there already is enough real food to feed everyone on the planet; there simply isn't access.

Preventing chronic diseases—for the first time in history responsible for the majority of deaths would not require massive public works programs like building water delivery or sewer systems but simply regulating the quality of our food and the quantity of the nonfood we allow ourselves to ingest. It is not a matter of technology or of miracles, but of policy. Minor inconveniences and infringements that benefit everyone—like seat belts, gun control, and limiting our "right" to smoke or drink—should take precedence over our "right" to kill ourselves and one another.

There is evidence not only in studies but also in the real world that public health policy measures can be successful. Why did the childhood obesity rate decline in such disparate places as New York City, Philadelphia, Mississippi, and California? It's simple: These places aggressively tackled dietary issues in schools and elsewhere.

In 2007, Mississippi's Healthy Students Act mandated 45 minutes per week of health education (home ec, anyone?) and limited the kinds of food and beverages sold in school vending machines. California banned sugary drinks in schools in 2009 and limited unhealthy snacks in 2007.

Philadelphia hasn't allowed soda or sugary drinks in vending machines in schools since 2004, and its schools no longer have deep-fryers; the Food Trust has pushed healthier food in corner stores. And New York has, among other things, banned trans fats from restaurants, made it easier for low-income people to shop at farmers' markets, and run a highly visible ad campaign that tells subway riders, for example, the number of miles they'd have to walk to account for that sugary drink.

Like Philadelphia, New York has come close to passing a soda tax, which has raised consciousness about the dangers of sugary drinks. As of this writing, Berkeley is the only city in the country that has passed a soda tax; others will likely follow.

These are dietary seat belts, and seat belts save lives. And only a jerk would say: "It's a slippery slope toward telling me what to do. If I want to ride without a seat belt, it's my right!"

When we see something, we should do something. The something we can all see is this: Eating badly—consuming unprecedented amounts of nonfood, like soda—causes obesity. Obesity brings about chronic disease. Chronic disease kills, wrecks lives, and wreaks havoc on our health care system and our economy. We have the power, collectively, to further reduce disease and improve longevity. Who's against that?

DECEMBER 18, 2012

11 Trillion Reasons

Here's a good line: "[U]nenlightened farm policy—with its massive subsidies for junk food ingredients—has played a pivotal role in shaping our food system over the past century. But that policy can readily be changed."

With the possible substitution of the word "might" for "can," this is pretty much an inarguable statement. It comes from "The $11 Trillion Reward: How Simple Dietary Changes Can Save Money and Lives, and How We Get There," a report produced by the Union of Concerned Scientists (U.C.S.).

That's a big number, $11 trillion, but even if it's off by 90 percent (it's difficult to put a value on lives), who's to scoff at a trillion bucks? In any case, this summary of current research, which contains the argument that even a tiny increase in our consumption of fruits and vegetables would have a powerful impact on health and its costs, agriculture, and the economy, is compelling.

About 750,000 United States deaths annually—a third of the total—result from cardiovascular disease, at a medical cost of about $94 billion. The report (and video based on it) maintains that if we upped our average intake of fruits and vegetables by a single serving daily—an apple a day, essentially—more than 30,000 of those lives would be saved (at an overall "value," according to the report, of $2.7 trillion). Each additional serving of fruit or vegetable would reduce mortality from cardiovascular disease by about 5 percent, to the point where if we all ate the recommended amounts of fruits and vegetables, we'd save more than 100,000 lives and something like $17 billion in health care costs. Note that this way of looking at things skips right by the obesity argument—which is fraught with controversy—and simply looks at the well-established notion that when you replace junk food with real fruits and vegetables you improve health.

This is not new, but the report—written by the U.C.S. agricultural econo-mist Jeffrey K. O'Hara—goes further, and points out that although Department of Agriculture (U.S.D.A.) dietary guidelines encourage all of us to eat sufficient fruits and vegetables to derive these benefits, that same department's agricul-tural policy encourages exactly the opposite—that is, damaging—behavior.

Thus we inevitably arrive at the infinitely negotiated Farm Bill, whose sub-sidies for commodity crops—soy, corn, and wheat are our chief concerns—directly promote the production of foods high in hyperprocessed carbohydrates and fats (for simplicity's sake, junk foods) and the kind of eating that is killing us. These policies come with many obvious direct costs, but also indirect ones. For by subsidizing the production of commodity crops we discourage the farm-ing of fruits and vegetables—the foods that promote health.

A main point of the report is that encouraging farmers to grow fruits and vegetables and sell them locally boosts public health. Therefore, U.C.S. wants to see programs that do just that, plus support research for noncommodity crops, subsidize the development of new outlets for locally grown food, and further encourage SNAP (food stamp) users to buy it.

A couple of other interesting points arise here. There's been a bit of back-lash about the new "L" word—local—by some economists, most pushers of in-dustrial agriculture and other skeptics, who scoff at the notion that adequate amounts of food can be grown locally. Putting aside the fact that "increasing re-gional production" is a more accurate way to describe what progressives in the food movement are advocating (few would argue that all food should be local), it's worth noting that with little government support the number of farmers' markets has quadrupled in the last 20 years, and that farm-to-school programs have grown from six in 2001 to more than 10,000 now.

Even if direct subsidies for fruits and vegetables—"specialty crops," as the U.S.D.A. almost mockingly calls them—were not forthcoming, a decrease in those subsidies for their competition would make these numbers even more impressive. Ending direct subsidies to what amounts to the enemies of good health makes so much sense that the U.C.S. report has received support from unexpected quarters. Eli Lehrer, president of the R Street Institute, a conserva-tive think tank, told me that "the central point of the report—that government agricultural subsidies contribute to worse health—is an excellent one, one that hasn't been made in this way."

Even Lehrer's critiques of the report are mild: "I can't say I hate any of the policy recommendations they make—they'd be better than what we're doing now—but if the subsidies are a problem, then replacing them with different types of subsidies isn't the solution."

My fear is that once you do away with subsidies for bad policies, the money is gone, and it will be difficult to get it back for the kind of programs U.C.S. advocates.

Still: I'll stand on common ground with anyone who wants to abandon subsidizing the growing of corn, Big Food's production of junk, and, ultimately, the undermining of public health. What happens afterward can hardly be worse.

That's the kind of thinking that Joshua Sewell, a senior policy analyst at the fiscally conservative Taxpayers for Common Sense, expressed as well: "There's a notion that we have to have spending on agriculture, but where's the money going and what are we getting out of it? The first step is to shift the paradigm and stop the harmful system we have now. The second step is to figure out the proper role of government, how to spend our money in a cost-effective manner: land grant universities should be doing research in the public interest, not corporate philanthropy."

It's not "cost-effective"—or, to put it more simply, smart—to subsidize the producers of food that makes us ill. They don't need it—they're already profitable, in part thanks to decades of subsidies—and there is no logic in helping corporations who are in the business of poisoning us to be more profitable. If government money is to go to agriculture, it should go to those farmers who are eager to grow the foods that will sustain us. What that's worth is inestimable.

AUGUST 6, 2013

The Right to Sell Kids Junk

The First Amendment to the Constitution, which tops our Bill of Rights, guarantees—theoretically, at least—things we all care about. So much is here: freedom of religion, of the press, of speech, the right to assemble, and more. Yet it's stealthily and incredibly being invoked to safeguard the nearly unimpeded "right" of a handful of powerful corporations to market junk food to children.

It's been reported that kids see an average of 5,500 food ads on television every year (sounds low, when you think about it), nearly all peddling junk. (They may also see Apple commercials, but not of the fruit kind.) Worse are the online "advergames" that distract kids with entertainment while immersing them in a product-driven environment. (For example: create your own Froot Loops adventure!)

And beyond worse: collecting private data, presumably in order to target children with personalized junk food promotions, which ask for permission to use your webcam to film you—without first verifying your age.

Remember: 17 percent of kids in the United States are obese (many more are nearly so), and though there is an argument that during the boom-and-bust periods of capitalism's development our genetic code has encouraged us to consume as many calories as possible, nowhere in our DNA is it written that we need to eat Big Macs, drink soda, or eat Twizzlers (much as I personally like the last of these). These cravings become habits as they are taught, encouraged, and reinforced by the marketing arm of Big Food, and the federal government appears powerless to change this. Here's where the First Amendment comes in.

I've written before about the government's pathetic attempt to nudge industry toward at least improving the nutritional profile of junk food advertising targeted at kids in the form of voluntary guidelines proposed by an interagency working group of the Federal Trade Commission, Centers for Disease Control and Prevention, Food and Drug Administration, and Department of Agriculture.

They suggested draft nutrition standards, and although the recommendations were absolutely nonbinding, the food and media industries erupted in opposition, forming an absurdly named lobbying group, the Sensible Food Policy Coalition ("Keep the government out of your kitchen!"), and seemingly managed to quash the release of a final report with actual recommendations.

Viacom, a member of the coalition, retained—that means paid—the renowned constitutional law scholar Kathleen M. Sullivan, who wrote that "government action undertaken with the purpose and predictable effect of curbing truthful speech is de facto regulation and triggers the same First Amendment concerns raised by overt regulation." On the flip side, an open letter signed by more than three dozen prominent legal scholars (who were not paid) countered that the guidelines "pose no threat to any rights guaranteed by the First Amendment."

It's easy to get lost in the Constitution and forget that we're talking about children being bombarded by propaganda so clever and sophisticated that it amounts to brainwashing, for products that can and do make them sick. Which brings me to this: an article published in the journal *Health Affairs* called "Government Can Regulate Food Advertising To Children Because Cognitive Research Shows That It Is Inherently Misleading." (Journals are not known for tabloid-like headlines, but this does get the point across.)

The authors, Samantha Graff, Dale Kunkel, and Seth E. Mermin, note that advertising was only granted First Amendment protection in the 1970s, when a series of decisions established that commercial speech deserves a measure of protection because it provides valuable information to the consumer, like the price and characteristics of a product.

"When the court extended the First Amendment to commercial speech," Graff told me, "it focused on how consumers benefit from unfettered access to information about products in the marketplace. But this notion has been twisted to advance the 'rights' of corporations to express their 'viewpoints' in the public debate—not only about their favored political candidates, but also about the wares they are hawking."

There is a legal test for judging whether commercial speech qualifies for protection under the First Amendment. Called the Central Hudson test, it says that such speech must be truthful and not "actually or inherently misleading." Since, as the authors point out, children under 12 cannot fully recognize and interpret bias in advertising, they're not equipped to make rational decisions about it. (Never mind that this is true of many adults also; that's a different story.) Based on relevant court decisions and scientific evidence, they contend, all advertising directed at children under 12 meets the legal definition of "inherently misleading," and therefore can be regulated by government.

They conclude that while regulating junk food advertising to kids may face all sorts of political opposition, like this bill to end "attack ads" against junk food, the First Amendment shouldn't stand in the way of tailored restrictions.

But although this kind of regulation may be constitutional, we're unlikely to see it any time soon, especially in an era of corporate "personhood." It's bad enough that kids are inundated with junk food ads on TV and online, but they're also seeing them in the schools they attend every day, and on the buses that take them there and back.

Nine states currently allow advertising on school buses, and 11 more, plus the District of Columbia, are considering it this year; nowhere is there language that prohibits food or beverage ads. Maine is the only state with a law prohibiting junk food marketing in schools, but according to a recent report, 85 percent of that state's schools visited were noncompliant, and most were wholly unaware of the law.

The U.S.D.A.'s much-improved school meals guidelines recently received kudos (even from me). But how in the name of the founding fathers can we justify feeding kids healthy food, while at the same time—and in the same place— encouraging them to eat junk?

Clearly, public schools need all the revenue they can get, but if the only way to sufficiently fund the schools is by undermining the nutrition of the kids who attend them, we'd better bring in more junk food ads, because we're going to have to pay for something else our kids will need:

Health care.

MARCH 27, 2012

¡Viva México!

Thanksgiving once marked the beginning of a season of belt-tightening, as fresh food became scarce. Now it launches a fury of gluttony—and it's not as if we're restrained at other times. Yet with obesity-associated Type 2 diabetes at record levels, it's widely agreed that we have to moderate this diet. Which means that, despite corporate intransigence, we have to slow the marketing of profitable, toxic, and addictive products masquerading as food.

It's logical to start with soda and other beverages sweetened with sugar or high-fructose corn syrup, which account for 7 percent of calories in the American diet, and many public health specialists have recommended a steep tax to reduce consumption. Ironically, France, which has a relatively low obesity rate, was the first to initiate a significant soda tax, and it seems to be reducing consumption but its soda drinking was relatively low to begin with. Now, however, it appears we're going to be able to judge such a tax, as well as the impact of a tax on junk foods, in a country known for obesity. This new tax is scheduled to be imposed in the new year, not in the supposedly progressive public health bastions of New York or San Francisco (though that city looks set to vote again on a soda tax in 2014), but in a country many Americans view as backward: Mexico.

Barring an unlikely court upset, the new year in Mexico will bring a national tax of one peso per liter—roughly 10 percent—on sugar-sweetened beverages and 8 percent on junk food. The legislation came about through a strong push by the Nutritional Health Alliance of 22 NGOs and networks representing some 650 nonprofits and grass-roots organizations, and an alignment of interests among President Enrique Peña Nieto, advisers in the Hacienda y Crédito

Público (the rough equivalent of the I.R.S.), and members of the opposition parties.

Industry will disagree, but sweetened beverages are generally acknowledged to be a direct cause of the obesity epidemic. The question, both in Mexico and in its immediate neighbor to the north (annual consumption in both countries is around 40 gallons per capita), has been how to curb it. Although President Obama murmured about a national soda tax in 2009, it never went beyond that, and attempts to establish taxes in various localities from New York to El Monte, Calif., have been defeated at the polls or otherwise blocked, always after huge industry campaigns.

The powerful Mexican soda and junk food industries were hardly asleep at the wheel this fall, and fear of losing their advertisers appears to have led major TV stations to refuse to run commercials advocating the tax. But several factors motivated Mexico's president and legislature, including the fact that among populous nations, Mexico recently passed the United States to become the world's most obese. Beyond that, there's an increasing awareness that Mexico's accelerating public health crisis could hurt its economy, and that only prevention would make practical the universal, single-payer health care system instituted last year.

In addition, agreed-upon financial reform meant that all unconventional funding sources had to be considered seriously; the tax is expected to bring in around $1 billion a year, and proponents of the tax had successfully linked its passage to a campaign assuring that purified drinking water would be made available in every school in the country. (Many believe that if there had been universal clean drinking water, the country would not have become so reliant on soda.) It may also be that the Peña Nieto government wanted to distinguish itself from its predecessors by claiming a new, highly visible place on the world stage.

Also critical to the new law was an agreement reached by the three major political parties, called "Pact for Mexico," which essentially committed them all to not blocking anything that a majority wanted; specifically, if the party in office and one of the other two major parties wanted to pass one of 95 reforms necessary for the country to progress the third party would not resist. In other words, the nation's future trumped partisan interests. (Americans may find this embarrassing, for obvious reasons.)

This has meant not only fiscal reform but more vigorous attempts to rein in corruption, break up monopolies in energy and communication, and aggressive public health moves, like the constitutional addendum of 2011 that guarantees all citizens "the right to nutritious, sufficient, and quality food." In fact the biggest takeaway may be that the government of the country with the world's 14th-largest gross domestic product has placed public health above the profits of an important industry.

Yes, this may have been a politically expedient calculation (and no, Mexico is hardly Nirvana), but the reality is that the regulation of an industry that needs regulation is happening. And there could hardly be a more important and legitimate role for government than attending to the health and well-being of its populace; we need not reflect too long on the inability or unwillingness of the government of the country with the world's largest economy to recognize this. (Equally embarrassing.)

Although the soda tax got most of the attention, other moves are also important. The junk food tax, first proposed at 5 percent but boosted to 8 when one senator argued that 5 percent didn't even cover the public expenditure on health problems caused by junk food, will use caloric density to define processed foods that are detrimental to health. The formula, which will exclude meat, dairy, and other "real" foods, would tax those foods that contain more than 275 calories per 100 grams, or just over three ounces. (For perspective: 100 grams of Snickers is about 500 calories; 100 grams of apple is approximately 50 calories.)

And although Mexico's Constitution forbids "earmarks"—tax revenues for specific purposes—there's at least preliminary agreement that much of the money from the new taxes be used for public health, including giving all schools drinking fountains that dispense purified water. (When asked if they were in favor of a soda tax, most Mexicans polled said no. When advocates linked the tax to obesity prevention, including clean water in schools, 70 percent were in favor. Soda tax campaigners, please note.) Especially in rural areas, people might end up using schools to get water for their homes, which would make it more likely that schools would be used to distribute subsidized fruits and vegetables, another goal of public health advocates.

Sugar (and by extension sugary beverages) is one of the three luxuries—along with tobacco and rum—described by Adam Smith as "extremely proper subjects of taxation"; it has proved to be the toughest to tax of the three. And although the soda tax is being hailed by supporters on both sides of the border (the American Heart Association said in a statement, "Mexico's effort provides an excellent starting point, but we need U.S. states and communities to enact the tax as well"), there is also wariness, because the tax is roughly half what research indicates to be the super-effectiveness threshold of about 20 percent. The peso-per-liter level is still meaningful, however; in fact, Femsa, Mexico's Coke bottler, has said it would pass on the tax by raising prices between 12 and 15 percent.

Still, it's difficult to be confident, especially since these taxes seem small against the overall challenge: significantly reducing consumption of sugar and controlling the marketing of junk food to kids. Furthermore, public health education is needed to turn around the culture of sugar, in which people may buy and drink sweet beverages despite higher costs and the presence of alternatives. When I visited Mexico City recently, tax advocates told me that the new moves made it clear that the previous administrations did nothing to prevent the obesity crisis (indeed, the next-to-last president was a former president of Coca-Cola Mexico). The new government has raised the stakes in defining a quality diet, recognizing that cheap calories are not sufficient and that real food is preferable to processed products.

Unlike the meaningless chant of "U.S.A.! U.S.A.!" (or the ridiculously chauvinistic "We're No. 1!"), ¡Viva México! actually means something: "Let Mexico Live!" (Or, more popularly, Long Live Mexico!)

But thanks largely to proximity (and NAFTA) Mexico has suffered more from adapting the standard American diet than any other country. Everyone, it seems, is surprised that these taxes are going forward. It would be fitting if they paved the way toward a saner diet, just as it would be both paradoxical and wonderful if the United States could follow its lead.

NOVEMBER 29, 2013

Bacteria 1, F.D.A. o

You may not have heard that the Maine-based grocery chain Hannaford issued a ground beef recall after at least 14 people were infected with an antibiotic-resistant strain of salmonella. After all, it's not much compared to the 76 illnesses and one death back in August that led Cargill to recall almost 36 million pounds of ground turkey products potentially contaminated with drug-resistant salmonella. The particulars get confusing, but the trend is unmistakable: our meat supply is frequently contaminated with bacteria that can't readily be treated by antibiotics.

A study earlier this year by a nonprofit research center in Phoenix analyzed 80 brands of beef, pork, chicken, and turkey from five cities and found that 47 percent contained Staphylococcus aureus, a bacteria that can cause anything from minor skin infections to pneumonia and sepsis, more technically called systemic inflammatory response syndrome (SIRS), and commonly known as blood poisoning—but no matter what you call it, plenty scary. Of those bacteria, 52 percent were resistant to at least three classes of antibiotics. So when you go to the supermarket to buy one of these brands of pre-ground meat products, there's a roughly 25 percent chance you'll consume a potentially fatal bacteria that doesn't respond to commonly prescribed drugs.

It's not like this is happening without a reason; the little germs have plenty of practice fighting the drugs designed to kill them in the industrially raised animals to which antibiotics are routinely fed. And although it's economical for producers to drug animals prophylactically, there are many strong arguments against the use of those drugs, including their declining efficacy in humans. (Economical, that is, as long as you don't count the cost of human lives and suffering or the actual dollars it costs to treat the disease. Once that's included, the cost to the U.S. health care system of treating such antibiotic-resistant infections in humans is estimated to be between $16 billion and $26 billion per year. But there's no reason for animal producers to care about that unless they're required to—or exhibit unusual levels of altruism.)

Probably you'd agree with the couple of people I described this situation to earlier this week, one of whom said something like, "Ugh, that's crazy," and the other simply, "They gotta do something about that!"

The thing is, "they" did. In 1977.

That's when the Food and Drug Administration, aware of the health risks of administering antibiotics to healthy farm animals, proposed to withdraw its prior approval of putting penicillin and tetracycline in animal feed. Per their procedure, the F.D.A. then issued two "notices of opportunity for a hearing," which were put on hold by Congress until further research could be conducted. On hold is exactly where the F.D.A.'s requests have been since your dad had sideburns.

Until last week, when the agency decided to withdraw them.

Not because the situation has gotten better, that's for sure; the agency is well aware that it's only gotten worse. A staggering 80 percent of the antibiotics sold in the U.S. are given to farm animals, mostly, as I said, prophylactically: the low-dose drugs help the animals fatten quickly and presumably help ward off diseases caused by squalid living conditions. The animals become perfect breeding grounds for bacteria to gain resistance to the drugs, and our inadequate testing procedures allow them to make their way into stores and our guts.

The F.D.A. knows all about this; in 2010 the agency issued a draft guidance proposing that Big Agriculture voluntarily (there's a non-starter for you) stop the use of low-dose antibiotics in healthy farm animals. "The development of resistance to this important class of drugs," the F.D.A. asserted, "and the resulting loss of their effectiveness as antimicrobial therapies, poses a serious public health threat." Good. Nice. But toothless.

So why would the F.D.A.—with full knowledge of the threat and a high-profile lawsuit by the Natural Resources Defense Council impelling them to finally address it—decide not to act?

In its announcement last week, the agency said that its "efforts will focus on promoting voluntary reform and the judicious use of antimicrobials in the interest of best using the agency's overall resources to protect the public health." What this means is that the F.D.A. has neither the budget nor the political support to mandate regulation.

That's true: the F.D.A. is consistently under-financed and increasingly unable to do its job, which is largely to protect the public health. It's worth noting that the F.D.A. is responsible for regulating antibiotics, but the Department of Agriculture (U.S.D.A.) oversees the actual animals that receive them. Why it's too much to ask for a single agency overseeing the production and health of animals is beyond me. It's also surprising that Congress recently increased the F.D.A.'s budget by an inadequate but better-than-nothing 3 percent. Most of that money is for implementing the Food Safety Modernization Act, a critical and long-overdue piece of legislation.

Here's the nut: The F.D.A. has no money to spare, but the corporations that control the food industry have all they need, along with the political power it buys. That's why we can say this without equivocation: public health, the quality of our food, and animal welfare are all sacrificed to the profits that can be made by raising animals in factories. Plying "healthy" farm animals (the quotation marks because how healthy, after all, can battery chickens be?) with antibiotics—a practice the EU banned in 2006—is as much a part of the American food system as childhood obesity and commodity corn. Animals move from farm to refrigerator case in record time; banning prophylactic drugs would slow this process down, and with it the meat industry's rate of profit. Lawmakers beholden to corporate money are not about to let that happen, at least not without a fight.

DECEMBER 27, 2011

E. Coli:
Don't Blame the Sprouts!

O ne hundred thousand E. coli can dance on the head of a pin; it may only take 50 to make you sick enough to die. Benign E. coli are everywhere, even in your own pink gut right now, and all E. coli can live on (or in) things as different as sprouts, burgers, and water. But if you were able to trace back far enough, their reservoir is most likely the gut of a mammal: a goat, a sheep, a deer, even a majestic elk or a dog. They're most often associated with cows.

The dangerous E. coli are called STEC (Shiga-toxin-producing E. coli, for the name of their horrific poison, and pronounced *ess-teck*). STEC usually migrate to food through direct or indirect contact with the contents of the animal's intestinal tract: dung, not to put too fine a point on it. Whether the growth or even origin of STEC—which have only been associated with human illness for 30 years—could have resulted in part from feeding cattle grain (as opposed to their natural grass), or was aided by industrial agriculture's unnecessary reliance on prophylactic antibiotics (a shameful story, but one that must wait), may never be known.

What is known is that if you keep STEC out of beef you partially solve the problem, and if you keep manure off other foods you partially solve the problem, too. It isn't easy, and it's never going to be foolproof, but these are the steps to take. If you're the cattle industry, you'd rather blame the whole thing on sprouts that were "somehow" contaminated. (Ban sprouts! No one really likes them anyway.) But blaming the sprouts is like blaming your nose for a virus-containing sneeze: That STEC came from somewhere, and in its history is an animal's gut.

Because they're grown in a warm, moist, gut-like environment, sprouts are an excellent vehicle for maintaining and maybe even reproducing STEC (indeed, so excellent that the Centers for Disease Control un-recommends them), but their involvement may never be proven.

Still, it's likely that when thousands of people were sickened by E. coli in Germany this year, they had eaten a vegetable that was contaminated in its handling: manure got into the growing or rinsing water; or it was on the hands of a picker; or it got dropped on a veggie by a bird, or brushed onto it by a wandering animal; or it was in a truck that took the sprouts to the packager, or some other innocent accident, the kind we must do our best to prevent, the kind that's magnified by combining huge lots of food from dozens of different sources and handling them all together. Remember, 50 STEC are enough to make you sick; one head of lettuce with a few hundred thousand bacteria, tossed together with a few tons of uncontaminated greens, then sold in thousands of packages, can mess up a lot of people.

Outbreaks of the deadly kinds of STEC—there are at least seven really toxic strains—are common enough. But these outbreaks are the tip of the iceberg; there are tens of thousands of "sporadic" cases from STEC every year in the United States alone, most of them unreported but no less deadly for that.

Although the U.S. has a pretty good track record when it comes to identifying and fighting STEC—thanks to much struggle on the part of lawyers and public health officials, and sound thinking in the U.S.D.A. and F.D.A.—we're falling way behind in preventing outbreaks like the current one, and we are even further behind in preventing the sporadic ones, those that get no headlines, remain unreported, and probably comprise the majority of cases. As is so common these days, a lack of funding and political will is the root of the problem.

The STEC that caused the infamous Jack in the Box outbreak of 1993 is formally called E. coli O157:H7. The U.S. has zero tolerance for that STEC, because in 1994—against the predictable protests of the meat industry—O157 was labeled an "adulterant," which means that any food in which it's discovered is recalled; happens all the time, though sometimes too late. There are, as I said, other STEC just as murderous, and we have a much more lenient policy about their presence in food: they're unregulated. Their presence in food is, legally speaking, just fine.

To slow the deadly effects of STEC, we need more and better basic and applied research to identify them and test for them. We also need more testing of water used for irrigation and washing; reduced animal intrusions; alert farm-workers (an aside: people tend to be more alert if they're more valued and less overworked and underpaid); and increased testing before people get sick and better reporting when they do get sick. (Less cow manure would help, but that isn't about to happen.) All of these steps take money.

Even more important, we need to immediately acknowledge that O157 is not the only deadly STEC out there (non-O157 STEC has been found in up to 6 percent of a random sampling of meat, and not just hamburger), an acknowl-edgment that—of course—the meat industry is unwilling to make. And we need to declare those other STEC as "adulterants" and get them out of the food supply to the best of our ability. The two agencies that can act on this are the U.S.D.A. and F.D.A., and both are hamstrung by budget policy (the F.D.A. needs more money for inspection; the House wants to give it less) and, of course, by the meat lobby and its allies.

Public health—arguably among the most important reasons for society's existence in the first place—has somehow become a "liberal" cause and there-fore unfashionable. But if the origin of these illnesses were bio-terrorism, money would be no object and even politics might be shunted aside. The fact is that a huge and powerful lobby would rather see a few thousand annual under-reported deaths and the occasional high-visibility outbreak than submit to fur-ther regulation and smaller profits. Especially if that outbreak is a world away. But next time it might not be.

JUNE 7, 2011

The F.D.A.'s Not-Really-Such-Good-News

That "good" news you may have read about the Food and Drug Administration's curbing antibiotics in animal feed may not be so good after all. In fact, it appears that the F.D.A. has once again refused to do all it could to protect public health.

Last week, the agency "requested" (that's the right word) that the pharmaceutical industry make a labeling change that, the F.D.A. says, will reduce the routine use of antibiotics in animal production. I'd happily be proven wrong, but I don't think it will. [Almost a year later, at this writing, antibiotic use in raising animals is up 8 percent.] Rather, I think we're looking at an industry-friendly response to the public health emergency of diseases caused by antibiotic-resistant bacteria, resistance that is bred in industrially raised animals.

You may know that 80 percent of antibiotics in the United States are given (fed, mostly) to animals. Why? Because the terrible conditions in which most of our animals are grown foster illness; give them antibiotics and illness is less likely. There is also a belief that "subtherapeutic" doses of antibiotics help animals grow faster. So most "farmers" who raise animals by the tens or hundreds of thousands find it easier to feed them antibiotics than to raise them in ways that allow antibiotics to be reserved for actual illness. (And yes, there are alternatives, even in industrial settings. Denmark raises as many hogs as Iowa and does it with far fewer antibiotics.)

You may also know that this overuse of antibiotics is leading to increasing bacterial resistance, that we're breeding an army of supergerms. This isn't theoretical: The Centers for Disease Control and Prevention estimates that 23,000 Americans die of illnesses related to antibiotic-resistant bacteria each year. Another two million are sickened. (Some experts say that these numbers are low.)

This makes resistant bacteria a greater health threat than AIDS, and there is talk by the C.D.C. of a post-antibiotic era.

The only solution, say most experts, is to stop the prophylactic use of antibiotics and use the drugs only to treat animals that are actually sick. (This is not news: Alexander Fleming, the discoverer of penicillin, feared microbial resistance and discussed it in his Nobel Prize speech of 1945.) Preventing this is an ostensible goal of the F.D.A., which itself predicted—in 1977—the very scenario in which overuse of antibiotics would lead to superbugs and, at that time, proposed to limit their use. But Congress got in the way and in the intervening years the agency appears to have been infiltrated by industry-friendly administrators who publicly write that "using these drugs judiciously means that unnecessary or inappropriate use should be avoided," yet manage to avoid enforcing these pronouncements.

The story of the last 36 years is one of inaction. The F.D.A. is already under a federal court order to "ensure the safety and effectiveness of all drugs sold in interstate commerce," and to withdraw drugs demonstrated to be unsafe—a court order the agency has appealed twice. One could see the new guidelines as little more than an attempt to convince the court to set aside its ruling.

Technically, reducing antibiotic use is simple. The science tells us it is the thing to do, the meat industry has the capability of designing animal-growing facilities that would foster less disease and, perhaps most important, the F.D.A. has the power to rule—not suggest—a complete ban of the use of antibiotics for growth promotion and disease prevention in livestock.

This last statement is contentious. Michael Taylor, the agency's deputy commissioner for foods and veterinary medicine (and—just in case you think the notion that there is a revolving door between the F.D.A. and the food industry is hyperbole—a former vice president for public policy at Monsanto), told me, "The approval of a new animal drug for specific indication is like the granting of a license; it applies to that company. There's a prescribed process for withdrawing that license . . . a very formal administrative process. We can't just issue a rule of general applicability that extinguishes their due process rights.

"We don't feel we have the legal authority," he continued, to do "what might be great to do from a public health policy standpoint. You'd have to show product by product that each is contributing" to a resistance problem. "This is a strategy to drive this to closure in the quickest way possible. We expect and hope folks will watch us closely."

We are talking about 287 different drugs, and Taylor says it might take "three or four years" to go through the process for each one. These guidelines, he says—which were developed with the cooperation of the industry (uh-huh)—will work faster.

But there are other ways of looking at the F.D.A.'s ability to regulate. These drugs fall into seven categories; nothing was preventing the agency, three or four years ago, from picking a drug from each category and beginning what Taylor calls "a very formal" process. Nothing prevents them from doing it now—simultaneously with their new guidelines   except, I would suggest, a desire to maintain a noncontentious relationship with Big Pharma and Big Food. As each drug, or category, was demonstrated to be unsafe, the process would become less cumbersome and something "great" might actually be done for public health.

It's not just me saying this.

Margaret Mellon, a lawyer and a senior scientist at the Union of Concerned Scientists, told me, "The agency can legally withdraw the label claims approvals if it can show that uses under the label circumstances are no longer safe in terms of resistance."

When I asked Representative Louise Slaughter—who happens to be a microbiologist, and is among the few in Congress with both the knowledge and spine to call out the F.D.A.—whether the agency had the authority to ban antibiotics for any use except direct treatment, she barely let me finish my question before exclaiming, "Of course they do."

And Robert Martin, a program director at the Center for a Livable Future at Johns Hopkins and a former director of the widely respected Pew Commission on Industrial Farm Animal Production, told me, "They have the authority to make these guidelines mandatory; the problem is that it's regulation by the consent of the regulated."

I could go on.

This in part explains why millions more are doomed to be sickened by the F.D.A.'s failures. You can blame Congress for inaction, too—shocking, I know. The Preservation of Antibiotics for Medical Treatment Act would require the F.D.A. to review its approvals of antibiotics and cancel them for antibiotics that help breed resistant bacteria; in fact it would put the burden of proof back on the companies, alleviating the workload and contentiousness Taylor seems intent on avoiding. (In fact, if the F.D.A. were truly interested in public health it would be out there lobbying for the passage of PAMTA.) Slaughter has introduced this act four times since 2007, and it's supported by almost everyone, but it hasn't passed. One wonders, though, since the F.D.A. is already under court order to do pretty much the same thing, whether even PAMTA would spur them on.

Instead, the F.D.A. has created a "road map for animal pharmaceutical companies to voluntarily revise the F.D.A.-approved use conditions on the labels of these products to remove production indications." No obligation. And no problem labeling those same drugs as disease-prevention vehicles, as long as those uses are "judicious and appropriate," says Taylor. Whether you call it growth promotion or disease prevention, the effects are likely to be on labels only, not on public health. (It seems to me that if you prevent disease you promote growth, and vice versa. It also seems to me that if you prevent disease by having healthy growing conditions you don't need to prevent it with antibiotics.)

And drug companies are O.K. with this new "guidance," because it's so benign it won't affect their bottom lines. In a *Wall Street Journal* piece, Jeff Simmons, the president of Eli Lilly's "animal-health division," was quoted as saying, "We do not see this announcement being a material event."

The F.D.A. says it "is asking animal pharmaceutical companies to notify the agency of their intent to sign on to the strategy within the next three months." (There are no provisions for noncooperation.) "These companies would then have a three-year transition process." In other words, drug companies have three months to "comply" with a voluntary plan to marginally change their labeling, and three years to implement that. Again, if they don't . . . sorry, there's no plan.

Strenuous oversight, huh? During which time industry can figure out how to increase the amount of antibiotics they sell, as long as they don't label them as growth-promoting. Yet Taylor insists that "this will make a difference for resistance."

In those three years, something like 69,000 Americans will have died from antibiotic-resistant bacterial diseases; many subsequent deaths may be preventable if rampant use of antibiotics is curbed now. But when insiders talk about the expected percentage decline in antibiotic use as a result of the F.D.A. recommendations, the smart money is on "zero." And when I asked Taylor, "How much do you anticipate routine antibiotic use declining in the next few years?" he answered, "It's a fair question but I don't have an answer for you—we need to work on that."

It's depressing. I root for the F.D.A. to do its job, but the power of industry and its anti-regulatory lobby adds up to an apparent unwillingness to put public health above all else. And by phasing this in over three years (by which time we'll have a new and possibly less supportive president), the agency has bought itself and the industry more time before bowing to the inevitable change in our horrific animal production system.

In fact, the worst thing about the new guidelines may be that they're seen as a first step, and as such rule out a more meaningful one. (Center for a Livable Future's Martin said to me, "My fear is now we won't see anything new for a decade.") It's bad news masquerading as good news. The F.D.A. is claiming, "We're controlling the use of antibiotics in animal production!" But it's more like Congress declaring, "We're raising the minimum wage!" and then appending ". . . by 10 cents an hour. And we'll review the impact of this monumental change in three years!"

I should point out that some of my favorite antibiotic-overuse critics are more optimistic, among them the former F.D.A. head David Kessler, who was quoted in these pages as saying, "This is the first significant step in dealing with this important public health concern in 20 years," and Laura Rogers, a director at the Pew Charitable Trusts, who told me, "These criteria represent a meaningful shift in the agency's public policy, and bode well for future action." ("That said," Rogers added, "we are concerned that antibiotics will still be used for disease prevention, possibly in place of growth promotion.")

Rogers is admirably diplomatic, but I agree more closely with Representative Slaughter, who wrote, "Sadly, this guidance is the biggest step the F.D.A. has taken in a generation to combat the overuse of antibiotics in corporate agriculture, and it falls woefully short of what is needed."

It's also worth noting that the F.D.A. has drafted (that means it's not even yet a recommendation) a "directive" that would require that veterinarians supervise antibiotic use. Make that final and make that mandatory—as the agency is threatening to do if these voluntary guidelines don't work—and we might be getting somewhere. But the best-case scenario is that within three years some or even all growth-promotion claims will have been dropped and the use of antibiotics will be approved by veterinarians—many of whom have jobs that will depend on approving just such uses. I see no reason to be encouraged. It may truly be worse than nothing, or it may simply be a delay we can ill afford.

Public safety is the F.D.A.'s job, and they're doing it badly. What's needed here is a drastic reduction in the use of antibiotics, now, and few people think these recommendations are going to do that. As the Union of Concerned Scientists' Mellon said to me, "This recommendation involves voluntarily giving up making money in the interest of public safety. Who does that in the United States? No one."

What can we do? Push for labeling, for one thing: "Raised without antibiotics" (period) is a label we could pay more attention to. And push our markets to carry more truly antibiotic-free meat, and buy it. Organic meat is another obvious solution. I'll get to strategies like these in another column. But as Slaughter said, "I'm persuaded now that the only thing we can do is get an outcry from the public." Make some noise, people.

DECEMBER 17, 2013

The 20 Million

Help wanted: Salary: $19,000 (some may be withheld or stolen). No health insurance, paid sick days, or paid vacation. Opportunity for advancement: nearly nil.

This job, or something much like it, is held by nearly 20 million people, 10 million of whom work in restaurants. They are the workers employed in producing, processing, and delivering our food, who have been portrayed in vivid and often dispiriting detail in a new report called "The Hands That Feed Us." Written by the Food Chain Workers Alliance, the report surveyed nearly 700 workers employed in five major sectors: production, processing, distribution, retail, and service.

The upshot: Our food comes at great expense to the workers who provide it. "The biggest workforce in America can't put food on the table except when they go to work," says Saru Jayaraman, co-founder of the Restaurant Opportunities Centers United (ROC-U).

Many people in the nascent food movement and in the broader "foodie" set know our farmers' (and their kids') names and what their animals eat. We practically worship chefs, and the damage done to land, air, and water by high-tech ag is—correctly—a constant concern.

Yet though you can't be a card-carrying foodie if you don't know the provenance of your heirloom tomato, you apparently can be one if you don't know how the members of your waitstaff are treated. We don't seem to mind or even notice that our servers might be making $2.13 an hour. That tip you debate increasing to 20 percent might be the difference in making the rent.

It's true that a bit of attention has been paid to farmworkers—with some good results, like mandated rest breaks, drinking water, toilet facilities, and even sometimes increased pay—and occasionally you read about the horrors of life in a slaughterhouse. But despite our obsession with food, the worker is an afterthought.

"The Hands That Feed Us," and the work being done on the ground by groups like ROC-U—which contributed to the report and helped create the Food Chain Workers Alliance in 2008—may signal the beginning of a change.

Take that $2.13 figure, the federal minimum wage for tipped workers. Legally, tips should cover the difference between that and the federal minimum wage (now a whopping $8). If they don't, employers are obligated to make up the difference. But that doesn't always happen, leaving millions of servers—70 percent of whom are women—taking home far less than the minimum wage.

Which brings us to the happily almost-forgotten Herman Cain. What's called the "tipped minimum wage"—that $2.13—once increased in proportion to the regular minimum wage. But in 1996, the year Cain took over as head of the National Restaurant Association (NRA), he struck a deal with President Bill Clinton and his fellow Democrats. In exchange for an increase in the regular minimum wage, the tipped minimum wage was de-coupled. The result: despite regular increases in the regular minimum wage, the tipped minimum wage hasn't changed since 1991.

Other disheartening facts: Only around one in eight jobs in the food industry provides a wage greater than 150 percent of the regional poverty level. More than three-quarters of the workers surveyed don't receive health insurance from their employers. (The Affordable Care Act has helped with that.) More than half have worked while sick or suffered injuries or health problems on the job, and more than a third reported some form of wage theft in the previous week. Not year: week.

There are societal considerations as well as moral ones: Food workers use public assistance programs (including, ironically, SNAP or food stamps) at higher rates than the rest of the United States workforce. And not surprisingly, more than a third of workers use the emergency room for primary care, and 80 percent of them were unable to pay for it. These are tabs we all pick up.

Senator Tom Harkin's (D-IA) proposed Rebuild America Act would raise the tipped minimum wage to $6.85 over five years (and the federal minimum wage to $9.80 by 2014), and allow more American workers to earn paid sick days. But Jayaraman (whose book, *Behind*, will be published next year) justifiably believes that these battles won't be won at a federal level without a massive shift in consumer thinking.

To that end, ROC-U produced a National Diner's Guide that rates restaurants based on how they treat their employees. (We have pocket guides for fish; finally, there's one for humans.)

Not surprisingly, most of the most notable abuses occur at the bigger companies. Remember Michelle Obama's spotlight on Walmart (the world's biggest food retailer) and the gigantic Darden Restaurant Company (which owns about 1,900 restaurants, including Olive Garden and Red Lobster), when she famously brokered deals with each that will ostensibly make their products "healthier"?

Well, both companies are known for labor abuses: Walmart for erratic and exhausting scheduling and hour-cutting, and Darden—highlighted in the ROC-U report—for low pay, no paid sick days, lack of breaks, and even racial discrimination. Those things tend not to come up when we're focusing on making our food system healthier.

On the other hand, Five Guys (with over 1,000 locations in the United States and Canada) evidently provides paid sick days and the opportunity for advancement.

Where would you rather eat?

That's a real question. If you care about sustainability—the capacity to endure—it's time to expand our definition to include workers. You can't call food sustainable when it's produced by people whose capacity to endure is challenged by poverty-level wages.

JUNE 12, 2012

Fast Food, Low Pay

In 2012, following the Black Friday protests by Walmart employees, 200 workers at 30 New York fast-food restaurants walked.

Not much happened immediately. There was press and vocal support from organized labor and the nascent food movement. But the strike didn't spread like wildfire.

Something else didn't happen, however: no one lost his job. And that was a huge deal.

As far as I can determine, only one worker was permanently terminated as a result of the many actions that have followed nationwide. Usually, the striking fast-food workers are escorted back to work by co-workers, clergy, union leaders, and even elected officials, who together insist that there be no retribution. That's worked.

And so a rapidly increasing number of food industry and other retail workers are now fighting for basic rights: halfway decent pay, a real work schedule, the right to organize, health care, paid sick days, vacations, and respect. Next week, organizers say, we'll see a walkout of thousands of workers at hundreds of stores in at least seven cities, including New York and Chicago.

Something is happening here, though exactly what isn't quite clear. Fast food was never a priority of organized labor—it's difficult to imagine a traditional union of four million fast-food workers in something like 200,000 locations—but dozens of organizations are now involved, including, to its credit, the Service Employees International Union, which is providing financing and counsel. The upshot: Workers with nothing to lose are demanding a living wage of $15 an hour, and gaining strength and confidence.

They don't have much else. Those making minimum wage and just above have less buying power than their peers did in the mid-'50s. Even business leaders are beginning to recognize that forcing workers onto food stamps is no way to sustain an economy—or a society. The chief executive of Costco, Craig Jelinek, for example, has endorsed President Obama's efforts to raise the minimum wage.

The movement found an unwitting ally when McDonald's offered its workers a sample personal budget that included such laughable features as the need for a second job and budget lines for "Heating" (zero) and "Health Insurance" ($20). Per month. (The company, which is worth $100 billion, give or take a few bucks, now says that heat costs $50 a month. But only if you speak English; the Spanish language site budgets heat at $30.) In the old days you could say: "So what? Those workers are all teenagers. They live at home." But the median age of today's fast-food worker is over 29, and many are trying to support families. One estimate claims that a family of four needs nearly $90,000 a year to get by in the nation's capital. That's six minimum-wage jobs. Explain to me, please, how you can be pro-family and anti-living-wage simultaneously? (Many Republicans in Congress seem to manage.)

We can afford to pay these workers: a petition titled "Economists in Support of a $10.50 U.S. Minimum Wage" estimates that McDonald's could recoup half the cost of such an increase simply by hiking the price of a Big Mac from $4 to $4.05. One item; 1 percent.

So the only reason this kind of outrage continues is that many ultrarich are denying the needs and suppressing the rights of our lowest paid workers. These people face huge odds, but equal challenges were overcome in both the 1930s and the 1960s by bold and sometimes "crazy" actions. There was mild government support then, and that's weaker now; but perhaps midterm elections will change that.

The recession killed 60 percent of $15- to $20-an-hour jobs, which should be the lowest-paying ones. Around 20 percent have returned, but the rest are being replaced by those paying less than $13 an hour. Thus median income for working-age households fell more than 10 percent from 2000 to 2010.

A vast majority of Americans are much closer in income to McDonald's workers than to corporate C.E.O.'s. Yet we tolerate the fact that one in seven of our fellow Americans live in poverty, with half of those people working tough jobs. Do we want to be part of that? Surely, better scenarios exist. And victory for the lowest-wage workers will have a positive impact on wages for everyone.

Six elements are affected by the way food is produced: taste, nutrition, and price; and the impact on the environment, animals, and labor. We can argue about taste, but it's clear that our production system—especially in the fast-food world—is flunking all the others. And if you think food is "cheap," talk to the people working in the fields, factories, and stores who can't afford it. Remember: no food is produced without labor.

Well-intentioned people often ask me what they can do to help improve our food system. Here's an easy one: When you see that picket line next week, don't cross it. In fact, join it.

JULY 25, 2013

The True Cost of Tomatoes

Mass-produced tomatoes have become redder, more tender, and slightly more flavorful than the crunchy orange "cello-wrapped" specimens of a couple of decades ago, but the lives of the workers who grow and pick them haven't improved much since Edward R. Murrow's revealing and deservedly famous "Harvest of Shame" report of 1960, which contained the infamous quote, "We used to own our slaves; now we just rent them."

But bit by bit things have improved some, a story that's told in detail and with insight and compassion by Barry Estabrook in his book, *Tomatoland*. We can actually help them improve further.

A third of our fresh tomatoes are grown in Florida, and much of that production is concentrated around Immokalee (rhymes with "broccoli"), a town that sits near the edge of the great "river of grass," or the Everglades, the draining of which began in the late 19th century, thus setting the stage for industrial agriculture. Immokalee is a poor (average annual per-capita income: $8,576), immigrant (70 percent of the population is Latino, mostly Mexican) working town, to the outsider at least a depressing community with few signs of hope.

The tomato fields of Immokalee are vast and surreal. An unplanted field looks like a lousy beach: the "soil," which is white sand, contains little in the way of nutrients and won't hold any water. To grow tomatoes there requires mind-boggling amounts of fertilizers, fungicides, and pesticides (on roughly the same acreage of tomatoes, Florida uses about eight times as many chemicals as California). The tomatoes are, in effect, grown hydroponically, and the sand seems useful mostly as a medium for holding stakes in place.

Most of the big purchasers, like Walmart and McDonald's, want firm, "slicing" tomatoes, because their destination is a burger or a sandwich, so the tomatoes are picked at what is called "mature green," which isn't mature at all but bordering on it. Tomatoes with any color other than green are too ripe to ship, and left to rot. The green tomatoes are gassed—"de-greened" is the chosen euphemism—to "ripen" them; the plants themselves are often killed with an herbicide to hasten their demise and get ready for the next crop.

The process, not to put too fine a point on it, is awful, but the demand is there—Florida ships about a billion pounds of tomatoes a year—and the main question has not been quality but fairness to the workers. (Estabrook profiles a successful Florida tomato farmer who's gone organic, but since it's inarguable that this is a locale and climate that's hostile to tomatoes in the first place, that can't be easy. Here's the reality: you're not going to get a billion pounds of good tomatoes out of Florida. Ever.)

Unlike corn and soy, tomatoes' harvest cannot be automated; it takes workers to pick that fruit. And not only have workers been enslaved, they have been routinely beaten, subject to sexual harassment, exposed to toxic chemicals (Estabrook mercilessly describes the tragic results of this) and forced to wait for hours to find out whether they have work on a given day. Oh, and they're underpaid.

One of the bright spots discussed in Estabrook's book is the Coalition of Immokalee Workers (CIW), founded in 1993. The CIW has two major goals: the first is to put the last nail in the coffin of slavery, a condition that sadly still exists not only among farmworkers but others. "And this," Laura Germino, who has worked on the campaign since its inception, said to me when I visited last month, "is not 'slavery-like,' or 'exploitation'—it's actual slavery, as defined by federal law." (There are super links around this issue on the anti-slavery campaign's website, and reading them is eye-popping.)

You've probably heard of the other goal, which is the CIW's Campaign for Fair Food; it's garnered as much attention as any labor struggle in the country in recent years, and more on the farmworker front than anything since the early work of Cesar Chavez and the United Farm Workers.

These outrages have been the CIW's focus, and the agreement they signed last November with the Florida Tomato Growers Exchange begins to address them: through the core "penny-a-pound" increase in the price wholesale purchasers pay, workers' incomes could go up thousands of dollars per year. The agreement also provides for a time-clock system in the fields, which has led to a shorter workday and less (unpaid) waiting time; portable shade tents for breaks (unbelievable that this didn't exist previously—I spent a half-hour in the open fields and began to melt); reduced exposure to pesticides; worker-to-worker education on rights; a new code of conduct for growers with real market consequences if workers' rights are violated; and more.

The breakthrough for the CIW came in 2005, when after enormous consumer pressure Yum! Brands, which controls Taco Bell, Pizza Hut, and KFC, signed the agreement. (And you know what? Good for them.) Since then, Subway, McDonald's, Burger King, the country's largest food service operators (Sodexo, Aramark, and Compass Group), and most supermarket chains have signed as well.

There are few places in the country where migrant and immigrant farmworkers are treated well; in Immokalee, at least, they're being treated better. Bit by bit.

JUNE 14, 2011

Legislating and Labeling

For all of the personal choices (like cooking, or supporting responsible farming) that can have a positive impact our food system, the kinds of sweeping changes that many of us hope to see can't be accomplished without decisive action at the top. Whether we know it or not, federal and local governments, which are all too often beholden to special interests, are largely responsible for deciding what we eat, because they refuse to restrict the behavior of producers and marketers, who then infallibly choose the most profitable—not the most healthful or even least destructive—paths. For example, we consume unknowable amounts of antibiotic residues because they're not labeled, dangerous quantities of sugary drinks because they're untaxed, and paltry amounts of fruits and vegetables because they're often not available.

The effects of these policies are visible everywhere, from supermarkets filled with indecipherable food labels, to doctors' offices and hospitals filled with patients suffering from diet-related diseases like obesity and diabetes. While attempts to regulate our food choices are often decried as "nanny-statism," the consequences of insufficient (or misguided) government intervention are significant.

Bad Food? Tax It,
and Subsidize Vegetables

What will it take to get Americans to change our eating habits? The need is indisputable, since heart disease, diabetes, and cancer are all in large part caused by the Standard American Diet. (Yes, it's SAD.)

Though experts increasingly recommend a diet high in plants and low in animal products and processed foods, ours is quite the opposite, and there's little disagreement that changing it could improve our health and save tens of millions of lives.

And—not inconsequential during the current struggle over deficits and spending—a sane diet could save tens if not hundreds of billions of dollars in health care costs.

Yet the food industry appears incapable of marketing healthier foods. And whether its leaders are confused or just stalling doesn't matter, because the fixes are not really their problem. Their mission is not public health but profit, so they'll continue to sell the health-damaging food that's most profitable, until the market or another force skews things otherwise. That "other force" should be the federal government, fulfilling its role as an agent of the public good and establishing a bold national fix.

Rather than subsidizing the production of unhealthful foods, we should turn the tables and tax things like soda, French fries, doughnuts, and hyperprocessed snacks. The resulting income should be earmarked for a program that encourages a sound diet for Americans by making healthy food more affordable and widely available.

The average American consumes 44.7 gallons of soft drinks annually. (Although that includes diet sodas, it does not include noncarbonated sweetened beverages, which add up to at least 17 gallons a person per year.) Sweetened drinks could be taxed at 2 cents per ounce, so a six-pack of Pepsi would cost $1.44 more than it does now. An equivalent tax on fries might be 50 cents per serving; a quarter extra for a doughnut. (We have experts who can figure out how "bad" a food should be to qualify, and what the rate should be; right now they're busy calculating ethanol subsidies.) Diet sodas would not be taxed.

Simply put: taxes would reduce consumption of unhealthful foods and generate billions of dollars annually. That money could be used to subsidize the purchase of staple foods like seasonal greens, vegetables, whole grains, dried legumes, and fruit.

We could sell those staples cheap—let's say for 50 cents a pound—and almost everywhere: drugstores, street corners, convenience stores, bodegas, supermarkets, liquor stores, even schools, libraries, and other community centers.

This program would, of course, upset the processed food industry. Oh well. It would also bug those who might resent paying more for soda and chips and argue that their right to eat whatever they wanted was being breached. But public health is the role of the government, and our diet is right up there with any other public responsibility you can name, from water treatment to mass transit.

Some advocates for the poor say taxes like these are unfair because low-income people pay a higher percentage of their income for food and would find it more difficult to buy soda or junk. But since poor people suffer disproportionately from the cost of high-quality, fresh foods, subsidizing those foods would be particularly beneficial to them.

Right now it's harder for many people to buy fruit than Froot Loops; chips and Coke are a common breakfast. And since the rate of diabetes continues to soar—one-third of all Americans either have diabetes or are pre-diabetic, most with Type 2 diabetes, the kind associated with bad eating habits—and because our health care bills are on the verge of becoming truly insurmountable, this is urgent for economic sanity as well as national health.

JULY 24, 2011

Justifying a Tax

At least 30 cities and states have considered taxes on soda or all sugar-sweetened beverages, and they're a logical target: of the 278 additional calories Americans on average consumed per day between 1977 and 2001, more than 40 percent came from soda, "fruit" drinks, mixes like Kool-Aid and Crystal Light, and beverages like Red Bull, Gatorade, and dubious offerings like Vitamin Water, which contains half as much sugar as Coke.

Some states already have taxes on soda—mostly low, ineffective sales taxes paid at the register. The current talk is of excise taxes, levied before purchase.

"Excise taxes have the benefit of being incorporated into the shelf price, and that's where consumers make their purchasing decisions," says Lisa Powell, a senior research scientist at the Institute for Health Research and Policy at the University of Illinois at Chicago. "And, as per-unit taxes, they avoid volume discounts and are ultimately more effective in raising prices, so they have greater impact."

Much of the research on beverage taxes comes from the Rudd Center for Food Policy and Obesity at Yale. Its projections indicate that taxes become significant at the equivalent of about a penny an ounce, a level at which three very good things should begin to happen: the consumption of sugar-sweetened beverages should decrease, as should the incidence of disease and therefore public health costs; and money could be raised for other uses.

Even in the current antitax climate, we'll probably see new, significant soda taxes soon, somewhere; Philadelphia, New York (city and state), and San Francisco all considered them last year, and the scenario for such a tax spreading could be similar to that of legalized gambling: once the income stream becomes apparent, it will seem irresistible to cash-strapped governments.

Currently, instead of taxing sodas and other unhealthful food, we subsidize them (with, I might note, tax dollars!). Direct subsidies to farmers for crops like corn (used, for example, to make now-ubiquitous high-fructose corn syrup) and soybeans (vegetable oil) keep the prices of many unhealthful foods and beverages artificially low. There are indirect subsidies as well, because prices of junk foods don't reflect the costs of repairing our health and the environment.

Other countries are considering or have already started programs to tax foods with negative effects on health. Denmark's saturated-fat tax is going into effect Oct. 1, and Romania passed (and then un-passed) something similar; earlier this month, a French minister raised the idea of tripling the value added tax on soda. Meanwhile, Hungary is proposing a new tax on foods with "too much" sugar, salt, or fat, while increasing taxes on liquor and soft drinks, all to pay for state-financed health care; and Brazil's Fome Zero (Zero Hunger) program features subsidized produce markets and state-sponsored low-cost restaurants.

Putting all of those elements together could create a national program that would make progress on a half-dozen problems at once—disease, budget, health care, environment, food access, and more—while paying for itself. The benefits are staggering, and though it would take a level of political will that's rarely seen, it's hardly a moonshot.

The need is dire: efforts to shift the national diet have failed, because education alone is no match for marketing dollars that push the very foods that are the worst for us. (The fast-food industry alone spent more than $4 billion on marketing in 2009; the Department of Agriculture's Center for Nutrition Policy and Promotion is asking for about a third of a percent of that in 2012: $13 million.) As a result, the percentage of obese adults has more than doubled over the last 30 years; the percentage of obese children has tripled. We eat nearly 10 percent more animal products than we did a generation or two ago, and though there may be value in eating at least some animal products, we could perhaps live with reduced consumption of triple bacon cheeseburgers.

Government and Public Health

Health-related obesity costs are projected to reach $344 billion by 2018—with roughly 60 percent of that cost borne by the federal government. For a precedent in attacking this problem, look at the action government took in the case of tobacco.

The historic 1998 tobacco settlement, in which the states settled health-related lawsuits against tobacco companies, and the companies agreed to curtail marketing and finance antismoking efforts, was far from perfect, but consider the results. More than half of all Americans who once smoked have quit and smoking rates are about half of what they were in the 1960s.

It's true that you don't need to smoke and you do need to eat. But you don't need sugary beverages (or the associated fries), which have been linked not only to Type 2 diabetes and increased obesity but also to cardiovascular diseases and decreased intake of valuable nutrients like calcium. It also appears that liquid calories provide less feeling of fullness; in other words, when you drink a soda it's probably in addition to your other calorie intake, not instead of it.

To counter arguments about their nutritional worthlessness, expect to see "fortified" sodas—à la Red Bull, whose vitamins allegedly "support mental and physical performance"—and "improved" junk foods (Less Sugar! Higher Fiber!). Indeed, there may be reasons to make nutritionally worthless foods less so, but it's better to decrease their consumption.

Forcing sales of junk food down through taxes isn't ideal. First off, we'll have to listen to nanny-state arguments, which can be countered by the acceptance of the anti-tobacco movement as well as a dozen other successful public health measures. Then there are the predictions of job loss at soda distributorships, but the same predictions were made about the tobacco industry, and those were wrong. (For that matter, the same predictions were made around the nickel deposit on bottles, which most shoppers don't even notice.) Ultimately, however, both consumers and government will be more than reimbursed in the form of cheaper healthy staples, lowered health care costs, and better health. And that's a big deal.

The Resulting Benefits

A study by Y. Claire Wang, an assistant professor at Columbia's Mailman School of Public Health, predicted that a penny tax per ounce on sugar-sweetened beverages in New York State would save $3 billion in health care costs over the course of a decade, prevent something like 37,000 cases of diabetes, and bring in $1 billion annually. Another study shows that a two-cent tax per ounce in Illinois would reduce obesity in youth by 18 percent, save nearly $350 million, and bring in over $800 million in taxes annually.

Scaled nationally, as it should be, the projected benefits are even more impressive; one study suggests that a national penny-per-ounce tax on sugar-sweetened beverages would generate at least $13 billion a year in income while cutting consumption by 24 percent. And those numbers would swell dramatically if the tax were extended to more kinds of junk or doubled to two cents an ounce. (The Rudd Center has a nifty revenue calculator online that lets you play with the numbers yourself.)

A 20 percent increase in the price of sugary drinks nationally could result in about a 20 percent decrease in consumption, which in the next decade could prevent 1.5 million Americans from becoming obese and 400,000 cases of diabetes, saving about $30 billion.

It's fun—inspiring, even—to think about implementing a program like this. First off, though the reduced costs of healthy foods obviously benefit the poor most, lower prices across the board keep things simpler and all of us, especially children whose habits are just developing, could use help in eating differently. The program would also bring much needed encouragement to farmers, including subsidies, if necessary, to grow staples instead of commodity crops.

Other ideas: We could convert refrigerated soda machines to vending machines that dispense grapes and carrots, as has already been done in Japan and Iowa. We could provide recipes, cooking lessons, even cookware for those who can't afford it. Television public-service announcements could promote healthier eating. (Currently, 86 percent of food ads now seen by children are for foods high in sugar, fat, or sodium.)

Money could be returned to communities for local spending on gyms, pools, jogging and bike trails; and for other activities at food distribution centers; for Meals on Wheels in those towns with a large elderly population, or for Head Start for those with more children; for supermarkets and farmers' markets where needed. And more.

By profiting as a society from the foods that are making us sick and using those funds to make us healthy, the United States would gain the same kind of prestige that we did by attacking smoking. We could institute a national, comprehensive program that would make us a world leader in preventing chronic or "lifestyle" diseases, which for the first time in history kill more people than communicable ones. By doing so, we'd not only repair some of the damage we have caused by first inventing and then exporting the standard American diet, we'd also set a new standard for the rest of the world to follow.

Some Progress on Eating and Health

For those concerned about eating and health, the glass was more than half full last week; some activists were actually exuberant. First, there was evidence that obesity rates among preschool children had fallen significantly. Then Michelle Obama announced plans to further reduce junk food marketing in public schools. Finally, she unveiled the Food and Drug Administration's proposed revision of the nutrition label that appears on (literally, incredibly) something like 700,000 packaged foods (many of which only pretend to be foods); the new label will include a line for "added sugars" and makes other important changes, too.

If the 43 percent plunge in obesity in young children holds true, it's fantastic news, a tribute to the improved Special Supplemental Nutrition Program for Women, Infants and Children (WIC), which encourages the consumption of fruits and vegetables; to improved nutrition guidelines; to a slight reduction in the marketing of junk to children; and probably to the encouragement of breastfeeding. Practically everyone in this country who speaks English or Spanish has heard or read the message that junk food is bad for you, and that patterns set in childhood mostly determine eating habits for a lifetime.

None of this happened by accident, and the lesson is that policy works.

The further limitations on marketing junk are more complicated. Essentially, producers won't be able to promote what they already can't sell (per new Department of Agriculture regulations), meaning that vending machines or scoreboards cannot encourage the consumption of sugar-sweetened beverages. (Promotion of increasingly beleaguered diet sodas would be allowed.)

Mrs. Obama's tendency to see the reformulation of packaged foods as an important goal is on display here: Snacks sold in schools (both in vending machines and out) will have to meet one of four requirements, like containing at least 50 percent whole grain or a quarter-cup of fruits or vegetables.

These proposed rules are better than nothing but filled with loopholes. Manufacturers will quickly figure out how to meet the new standards, and the improvements, though not insignificant, will not go far in teaching kids that the best snack is an apple or a handful of nuts. (One way to really clobber junk food would be to prevent companies from taking tax deductions on the marketing of unhealthy foods, a move that's in a bill sponsored by Congresswoman Rosa DeLauro of Connecticut, one that won't pass until we're in some kind of unforeseeable new era.)

Still. It beats calling ketchup a vegetable.

The label change is huge. Yes: It could be huge-er. Yes: It's long overdue. Yes: It may be fought by industry and won't be in place for a long time. And yes: The real key is to be eating whole foods that don't need to be labeled.

But by including "added sugars" on the label, the F.D.A. is siding with those who recognize that science shows that added sugars are dangerous. "This is an acknowledgment by the agency that sugar is a big problem," says the former F.D.A. commissioner David Kessler, who presided over the development of the last label change, 20 years ago. "It will allow the next generation to grow up with far more awareness."

Big Food has long maintained that it doesn't matter where sugar or indeed calories come from—that they're all the same. But "added sugars" declares the industry's strategy of pumping up the volume on "palatability," making ketchup, yogurt, and granola bars, for example, as sweet and high-caloric as jam, ice cream, and Snickers. Added sugar turns sparkling water into soda and food-like objects into candy. Added sugar, if you can forgive the hyperbole, is the enemy. This is not to say you shouldn't eat a granola bar, but if you know what's in it you're less likely to think of it as "health food."

There are a couple of other significant changes, including more realistic "serving sizes" (a serving of ice cream will now be a more realistic cup instead of a half-cup, for example), the deletion of the "calories from fat" line, which recognizes that not all fats are "bad," and some changes in daily recommended values for various nutrients.

Mrs. Obama, who is sometimes seen (by me among many others) as overly industry-friendly, was behind the push for these changes, or at least highly supportive of them. And she deserves credit: It's a victory, and no one on the progressive side of this struggle should see it as otherwise.

The label is hardly messianic. In fact, the F.D.A. tacitly acknowledges this by offering an alternative, stronger label, which approaches the kind of "traffic light" labeling I've advocated for, and which there's evidence to support. The alternative has four sections, including "Avoid Too Much" and "Get Enough"; the first includes added sugars and trans fat, for example, and the second, fiber and vitamin D.

Michael Taylor, the F.D.A.'s deputy commissioner for foods and veterinary medicine—and the guy who supervised the new label's development—told me that the alternative label is essentially a way to further "stimulate comments." It may be that it's also a demonstration of the agency's will, designed to show industry how threatening things could get so Big Food will swallow the primary label without much complaint.

Although the ultimate decision is the F.D.A.'s, the Grocery Manufacturers' Association statement last week said in part, "It is critical that any changes are based on the most current and reliable science." These are, and marketers are going to have a tough time claiming otherwise. In other words, we're going to see some form of new and stronger label, period.

Introducing the label, Mrs. Obama said, "Our guiding principle here is very simple: that you as a parent and a consumer should be able to walk into your local grocery store, pick up an item off the shelf, and be able to tell whether it's good for your family."

This label moves in that direction, but it could be much more powerful. Kessler would like to see a pie chart on the front of the package: "That would help people know what's real food and what's not." Michael Pollan also suggests front-of-the-box labeling: "I think the U.K. has the right idea with their stoplight panel on the front of packages; only a small percentage of shoppers get to the nutritional panel on the back." And the N.Y.U. nutrition professor Marion Nestle (who called this label change "courageous") says, "A recommended upper limit for added sugars would help put them in context; I'd like to see that set at 10 percent of calories or 50 grams (200 calories) in a 2,000-calorie diet." I've written about my own dream label (see page 210), which contains categories that probably won't be considered for another 10 years—if ever.

What else is wrong? The label covers a lot of food, but it has no effect on restaurant food, takeout, most prepared food sold in bulk (do you have any idea what's in that fried chicken at the supermarket deli counter, for example?), or alcohol.

The Obama administration and the F.D.A. have made a couple of moves here that might be categorized as bold, but they could have done so three or four years ago; these are regulations that can be built upon, and do not require Congressional approval. But by the time they're in effect it may be too late for this administration to take them to the next level.

In short, it's not a case of too-little-too-late but one of "it could've been more and happened sooner."

But that's looking backward instead of forward. If we see a decline in obesity rates, more curbs on food marketing, and greater transparency in packaged food, that's progress. Let's be thankful for it, then get back to work pushing for more.

MARCH 4, 2014

Why Do GMOs
Need Protection?

G enetic engineering in agriculture has disappointed many people who once had hopes for it. Excluding, of course, those who've made money from it, appropriately represented in the public's mind by Monsanto. That corporation, or at least its friends, recently managed to have an outrageous rider slipped into the 587-page funding bill Congress sent to President Obama.

Incredibly, it was done anonymously. No member of Congress has taken responsibility.

The rider essentially prohibits the Department of Agriculture from stopping production of any genetically engineered crop once it's in the ground, even if there is evidence that it is harmful.

That's a pre-emptive Congressional override of the judicial system, since it is the courts that are most likely to ask the U.S.D.A. to halt planting or harvest of a particular crop. President Obama signed the bill last week (he kind of had to, to prevent a government shutdown) without mentioning the offensive rider he might have, despite the gathering of more than 250,000 signatures protesting the rider by the organization Food Democracy Now! Nor did he mention another horrendous House-inserted provision that gives increased market power to our three largest meatpacking corporations at the expense of small farmers and ranchers, and hogties U.S.D.A. attempts to put the brakes on the worst abuses of big meatpackers.

The override is unnecessary as well as disgraceful, because the U.S.D.A. is already overly supportive of genetically engineered crops. When a court tried to stop the planting of genetically engineered beets a couple of years ago pending adequate study, the U.S.D.A. allowed it. And the secretary of agriculture, Tom

Vilsack—who, in fairness, does not seem happy about the rider but was power-less to stop it—was quoted as saying, "With the seed genetics today that we're seeing, miracles are occurring every single growing season."

True enough. But "seed genetics" refers not only to genetically engineered seeds but to seeds whose genetics have been altered by conventional means, like classical breeding. In fact, as I said up top, genetic engineering, or, more properly, transgenic engineering—in which a gene, usually from another species of plant, bacterium, or animal, is inserted into a plant in the hope of positively changing its nature—has been disappointing.

In the nearly 20 years of applied use of G.E. in agriculture there have been two notable "successes," along with a few less notable ones. (This from a technology that its advocates promised would be revolutionary, a technology that some believe is our only hope of increasing yields quickly enough to "feed humanity" later this century.) These are crops resistant to Monsanto's Roundup herbicide (Monsanto develops both the seeds and the herbicide to which they're resistant) and crops that contain their own insecticide. The first have already failed, as so-called superweeds have developed resistance to Roundup, and the second are showing signs of failing, as insects are able to develop resistance to the inserted Bt toxin—originally a bacterial toxin—faster than new crop variations can be generated.

Nothing else in the world of agricultural genetic engineering even comes close to the "success" of these two not-entirely-successful creations. Furthermore, at least in these cases, their pattern of success (and high profits) followed by failure was inevitable.

Don't take my word for it. Let me summarize extensive conversations I've had with Doug Gurian-Sherman, a senior scientist and plant pathologist at the Union of Concerned Scientists: Roundup Ready seeds allowed farmers to spend less time and energy controlling weeds. But the temporary nature of the gains was predictable: "There was no better way to create weeds tolerant to glyphosate (Roundup) than to spray all of them intensively for a few years," Gurian-Sherman told me. "And that's what was done."

The result is that the biggest crisis in monocrop agriculture—something like 90 percent of all soybeans and 70 percent of corn is grown using Roundup Ready seed—lies in glyphosate's inability to any longer provide total or even predictable control, because around a dozen weed species have developed resistance to it. "Any ecologist would have predicted this, and many did," Gurian-Sherman said.

In the case of seeds containing the Bt toxin, insect resistance took longer to develop because breeders, knowing that insects evolve faster than new crop species can normally be generated, have deployed several variations of the Bt toxin in an effort to reduce the "selection pressure." But, says Gurian-Sherman, "We're starting to see that resistance now."

Aside from the shame of Congress, there is another important issue here. Many steps could be taken right now to improve yields while diminishing the need for herbicides and pesticides, including sophisticated rotational systems, targeted applications of chemicals, and other methods tested and demonstrated in the U.S.D.A./Iowa State University Marsden Farm study (about which I wrote last year). Acknowledging that—and recognizing that, at least for now, classical breeding methods remain superior to genetic engineering for whole crop improvement—is not the same thing as making inflated claims about the hazards of genetic engineering to human health, as some opponents of genetic engineering have taken to doing.

There is far from any scientific consensus on this, because there's currently little or no reliable evidence that food manufactured with ingredients from genetically engineered plants is directly harmful to humans. On the other hand, there has been no monitoring of humans for harm, so the very often heard claim by many G.E. advocates that the technology has harmed no one is, says Gurian-Sherman, "flat out wrong scientifically." That's not the same thing as saying that the potential isn't there for novel proteins and other chemicals to generate unexpected problems, which is why we need strict, effective testing and regulatory systems.

It's also why the pre-emptive "biotech rider" is such an insult: Congress is (again) protecting corporations from the public interest. This is all the more reason that food derived from genetically modified organisms should be so labeled, especially since the vast majority of Americans want it to be.

Still, we should abhor the use of genetically engineered seeds without adequate testing, and protest against hijacking the Constitution to guarantee the "right" to unregulated use of genetically engineered seeds. It's smart to prudently explore the possible benefits and uses of genetically engineered materials in agriculture, and to deploy them if and when they're proven to be a) safe (otherwise, no) and b) beneficial to society at large (otherwise, why bother?). I don't believe that any G.E. materials have so far been proven to be either of these things, and therefore we should proceed cautiously.

We should also note that far less expensive—sometimes 100 times less expensive—conventional breeding techniques have outstripped genetic engineering techniques over the last 20 years, during which G.E. techniques have gotten far more publicity. (Conventionally bred drought resistance has raised yields around 30 percent in the last 30 years; Monsanto's drought-resistant corn, says Gurian-Sherman, promises at most a 6 percent increase, and that only in moderate drought.) We're using more pesticides than ever (something like 400 million pounds in the last 15 years), and net yields from applied genetic engineering in the United States are only a bit higher (and then only in mono-crop systems) than net yields from seeds developed using more conventional techniques.

All of this explains why producers of genetically engineered seeds feel they need protection. (One can only hope that this is temporary, since the rider expires at the end of this fiscal year; though it's hard to see it going away without a whole lot of noise.) Their technology is not that great (did Polaroid, or Xerox, or Microsoft need protection?) and their research costs are high. They need another home run like Roundup Ready crops—serious drought tolerance would be an example—yet there isn't one in sight.

Genetic engineering has its problems. Like nuclear power, it may someday become safe and productive or—again like nuclear power—it may become completely unnecessary. Our job as citizens is to support the production of energy and food by the most sustainable and least damaging methods scientists can devise. If that's genetic engineering, fine. But to date it hasn't been; in fact, the technology has been little more than an income-generator for a few corporations desperate to see those profits continue regardless of the cost to the rest of us, or to the environment.

APRIL 2, 2013

Why Aren't GMO Foods Labeled?

If you want to avoid sugar, aspartame, trans fats, MSG, or just about anything else, you read the label. If you want to avoid GMOs—genetically modified organisms—you're out of luck. They're not listed. You could, until now, simply buy organic foods, which by law can't contain more than 5 percent GMOs. Now, however, even that may not work.

This year, the U.S. Department of Agriculture has approved three new kinds of genetically engineered (G.E.) foods: alfalfa (which becomes hay), a type of corn grown to produce ethanol, and sugar beets. And the approval by the Food and Drug Administration of a super-fast-growing salmon—the first genetically modified animal to be sold in the U.S., but probably not the last—may not be far behind.

It's unlikely that these products' potential benefits could possibly outweigh their potential for harm. But even more unbelievable is that the F.D.A. and the U.S.D.A. will not require any of these products, or foods containing them, to be labeled as genetically engineered, because they don't want to "suggest or imply" that these foods are "different." (Labels with half-truths about health benefits appear to be O.K., but that's another story.)

They are arguably different, but more important, people are leery of them. Nearly an entire continent—it's called Europe—is so wary that G.E. crops are barely grown there and there are strict bans on imports (that policy is still in danger). Furthermore, most foods containing more than 0.9 percent GMOs must be labeled.

G.E. products may grow faster, require fewer pesticides, fertilizers, and herbicides, and reduce stress on land, water, and other resources; they may be more profitable to farmers. But many of these claims are in dispute, and advances in conventional agriculture, some as simple as drip irrigation, may achieve these same goals more simply. Certainly conventional agriculture is more affordable for poor farmers, and most of the world's farmers are poor. (The surge in suicides among Indian farmers has been attributed by some, at least in part, to G.E. crops, and it's entirely possible that what's needed to feed the world's hungry is not new technology but a better distribution system and a reduction of waste.)

To be fair, two of the biggest fears about G.E. crops and animals—their potential to provoke allergic reactions and the transfer to humans of antibiotic-resistant properties of GMOs—have not come to pass, and I don't believe they're likely to. (I could be wrong, of course.) But there has been cross-breeding of natural crops and species with those that have been genetically engineered, and when ethanol corn cross-pollinates feed corn, the results could degrade the feed corn; when G.E. alfalfa cross-pollinates organic alfalfa, that alfalfa is no longer organic; if a G.E. salmon egg is fertilized by a wild salmon, or a transgenic fish escapes into the wild and breeds with a wild fish . . . it's not clear what will happen.

Cross-breeding is guaranteed with alfalfa and likely with corn. (The U.S.D.A. claims to be figuring out ways to avoid this happening, but by then the damage may already be done.) And the organic dairy industry is going to suffer immediate and frightening losses when G.E. alfalfa is widely grown, since many dairy cows eat dried alfalfa (hay), and the contamination of organic alfalfa means the milk of animals fed with that hay can no longer be called organic. Likewise, when feed corn is contaminated by G.E. ethanol corn, the products produced from it won't be organic. (On the one hand, the U.S.D.A. joins the F.D.A. in not seeing G.E. foods as materially different; on the other it limits the amount found in organic foods. Hello? Guys? Could you at least pretend to be consistent?)

The subject is unquestionably complex. Few people outside of scientists working in the field—myself included—understand much of anything about gene altering. Still, an older ABC poll found that a majority of Americans believe that GMOs are unsafe, even more say they're less likely to buy them, and a more recent CBS/NYT poll found a whopping 87 percent—you don't see a poll number like that too often—wants them labeled. This is as nonpartisan as an issue gets.

In the long run, genetic engineering may prove to be useful. Or not. The science is adolescent at best; not even its strongest advocates can guarantee that there aren't hidden dangers. So consumers are understandably cautious, and whether that's justified or paranoid, it would seem we have a right to know as much as Europeans do.

Even more than questionable approvals, it's the unwillingness to label these products as such—even the G.E. salmon will be sold without distinction—that is demeaning and undemocratic, and the real reason is clear: producers and producer-friendly agencies correctly suspect that consumers will steer clear of G.E. products if they can identify them. Which may make them unprofitable—and that might not be a bad thing. If a decline in profitability of GMOs were to lead to a greater focus on research in all fields of agriculture, that would be a plus. One could also argue that if GMOs were to become less profitable, their producers would be more cooperative with others in the field. You cannot, for example, analyze or research genetically modified seeds without express permission from their creator.

A majority of our food already contains GMOs, and there's little reason to think more isn't on the way. It seems our "regulators" are using us and the environment as guinea pigs, rather than demanding conclusive tests. And without labeling, we have no say in the matter whatsoever.

FEBRUARY 1, 2011

Leave "Organic" Out of It

The ever-increasing number of people working to improve the growing, processing, transporting, marketing, distributing, and eating of food must think through our messages more thoroughly and get them across more clearly. I don't pretend to have all the answers, but I can say that a couple of buzzwords represent issues that are far more nuanced than we often make them appear. These are "organic" and "GMOs" (genetically modified organisms).

I think we—forward-thinking media, progressives in general, activist farmers, think-tank types, nonprofiteers, everyone who's battling to create a better food system—often send the wrong message on both of these. If we understand and explain them better it'll be more difficult for us to be discredited (or, worse, dismissed out of hand), and we'll have more success moving intelligent comments on these important issues into the mainstream.

Let's start with "organic." The struggle to raise more food in more sustainable ways is as important as any, including the fight to slow climate change. (They're related, of course.) But more sustainable does not mean "pure," and organic often generates unreasonable expectations. Many experts are now using the term "agro-ecological," which has the disadvantage of being unusable in casual conversation—why not just say, "We want to make crop production better?" Because we can improve industrial agriculture more quickly and easily than we can convert the whole system to "organic," which is never going to happen. Unless, of course, we run out of cheap fossil fuel and have to stop moving chemicals and food around the globe willy-nilly.

Furthermore, there's a very real difference between eating better and growing better. I can eat better starting right now, and it has nothing—zero—to do with shopping at Whole Foods or eating organically. It has to do with eating less junk, hyperprocessed food, and industrially raised animal products. The word "organic" need not cross my lips.

Often I'm engaged in a discussion where I say precisely that: Eat more plants, try to wipe out junk food from your diet, cut back on industrially produced animal products, and so on. Inevitably, someone asks, "What if I can't afford to buy organic?" Or, "What if I can't afford to shop at Whole Foods?"

Let's encourage people to eat real food, which for most people will mean eating better. This is affordable for nearly everyone in the United States. For most people, eating better is mostly about will and skill. Those are not small items, but they're much more easily dealt with than changing industrial agriculture. Yes, there are people who are too poor to afford real food; but that's an issue of justice, the right to food, and fair wages—not of whether the food is organic.

Eating organic food is unquestionably a better option than eating nonorganic food; at this point, however, it's a privilege. But that doesn't make it a deal-breaking matter. Reducing the overload of synthetic chemicals and drugs in agriculture and the environment is a huge issue, as is eating better, but neither necessitates "going organic."

Then there are GMOs: OMG (the palindrome is irresistible). Someone recently said to me, "The important issues are food policy, sustainability, and GMOs." That's like saying, "The important issues are poverty, war, and dynamite." GMOs are cogs in industrial agriculture, the way dynamite is in war; take either away, and you have solved virtually nothing.

By themselves and in their current primitive form, GMOs are probably harmless; the technology itself is not even a little bit nervous making. (Neither we nor plants would be possible without "foreign DNA" in our cells.) But to date GMOs have been used by companies like Monsanto to maximize profits and further remove the accumulated expertise of generations of farmers from agriculture; in those goals, they've succeeded brilliantly. They have not been successful in moving sustainable agriculture forward (which is relevant because that was their claim), nor has their deployment been harmless: It's helped accelerate industrial agriculture and its problems and strengthened the positions of unprincipled companies.

But the technology itself has not been found to be harmful, and we should recognize the possibility that the underlying science could well be useful (as dynamite can be useful for good), particularly with greater public investment and oversight.

Let's be clear: Biotech in agriculture has been overrated both in its benefits and in its dangers. And by overrating its dangers, the otherwise generally rational "food movement" allows itself to be framed as "anti-science."

If anti-GMO activists were successful in banning GMOs, we'd still have industrial agriculture, along with its wholesale environmental degradation and pollution, labor abuse, and overproduction of ingredients for the junk food diet.

What about labeling? I'm in favor of transparency—I want to know what's in my food—and labeling GMOs may well be the thin end of the wedge. But that GMOs are in the forefront of the battle for transparency is perhaps unfortunate, since they play on irrational fears and are far less worrisome than the intensive and virtually unregulated use of antibiotics and agricultural chemicals.

Maybe all I'm saying here is this: There are two important struggles in food: One is for sustainable agriculture and all that it implies—more respect for the earth and those who live on it (including workers), more care in the use of natural resources in general, more consideration for future generations. The other is for healthier eating: a limit to outright lies in marketing "food" to children, a limit on the sales of foodlike substances, a general encouragement for the eating of real food.

Both sustainability and healthier eating affect us. Very few people can avoid struggling daily with the avalanche of bad food and the culture and propaganda surrounding it. Near-hysteria or simple answers lead to unachievable situations and nonsolutions. More effective would be shifting the food culture, the relevant business models, and public policies—a gradual and concerted movement toward making production and consumption simply "better." That is what the good food movement should be about.

MAY 6, 2014

My Dream Food Label

What would an ideal food label look like? By "ideal," I mean from the perspective of consumers, not marketers.

NUTRITION	●	● ●	● ●	●	**12 / 15**
FOODNESS	●	● ●	● ●	○	
WELFARE	●	● ●	● ●	●	

Right now, the labels required on food give us loads of information, much of it useful. What they don't do is tell us whether something is really beneficial, in every sense of the word. With a different set of criteria and some clear graphics, food packages could tell us much more.

Even the simplest information—a red, yellow, or green "traffic light," for example—would encourage consumers to make healthier choices. That might help counter obesity, a problem all but the most cynical agree is closely related to the consumption of junk food.

Of course, labeling changes like this would bring cries of hysteria from the food producers who argue that all foods are fine, although some should be eaten in moderation. To them, a red traffic-light symbol on chips and soda might as well be a skull and crossbones. But traffic lights could work: indeed, in one study, sales of red-lighted soda fell by 16.5 percent in three months.

A mandate to improve compulsory food labels is unlikely any time soon. Front-of-package labeling is sacred to big food companies, a marketing tool of the highest order, a way to encourage purchasing decisions based not on the truth but on what manufacturers would have consumers believe.

So think of the creation of a new food label as an exercise. Even if some might call it a fantasy, the world is moving this way. Traffic-light labeling came close to passing in Britain, and our own Institute of Medicine is proposing something similar. The basic question is, how might we augment current food labeling (which, in its arcane detail, serves many uses, including alerting allergic people to every specific ingredient) to best serve not only consumers but all contributors to the food cycle?

As desirable as the traffic light might be, it's merely a first step toward allowing consumers to make truly enlightened decisions about foods. Choices based on dietary guidelines are all well and good—our health is certainly an important consideration—but they don't go nearly far enough. We need to consider the well-being of the earth (and all that that means, like climate, and soil, water, and air quality), the people who grow and prepare our food, the animals we eat, the overall wholesomeness of the food—what you might call its "foodness" (once the word "natural" might have served, but that's been completely co-opted), as opposed to its fakeness. ("Foodness" is a tricky, perhaps even silly word, but it expresses what it should. Think about the spectrum from fruit to Froot Loops or from chicken to Chicken McNuggets and you understand it.) These are considerations that even the organic label fails to take into account.

Beyond honest and accurate nutrition and ingredient information, it would serve us well to know at a glance whether food contains trans fats; residues from hormones, antibiotics, pesticides, or other chemicals; genetically modified ingredients; or indeed any ingredients not naturally occurring in the food. It would also be nice to be able to quickly discern how the production of the food affected the welfare of the workers and the animals involved and the environment. Even better, it could tell us about its carbon footprint and its origins.

A little of this is covered by the label required for organic food. Some information is voluntarily being provided by producers—though they're most often small ones—and retailers like Whole Foods. But only when this kind of information is required will consumers be able to express preferences for health, sustainability, and fairness through our buying patterns.

Still, one can hardly propose covering the front of packages with 500-word treatises about the product's provenance. On the other hand, allowing junk food to be marketed as healthy is unacceptable, or at least would be in a society that valued the rights of consumers over those of the corporation. (The "low-fat" claim is the most egregious—plenty of high-calorie, nutritionally worthless foods are in fact fat-free—but it's not alone.)

All of this may sound like it's asking a lot from a label, but creating a model wasn't that difficult. For several months, I worked with Werner Design Werks of St. Paul to devise a food label that, at perhaps little more than a glance (certainly in less than 10 seconds), can tell a story about three key elements of any packaged food and can provide an overall traffic-light-style recommendation or warning.

How such a labeling system could be improved, which agency would administer it (it's now the domain of the F.D.A.), which producers would be required to use it, whether foods should carry quick-response codes that let your phone read the package and link to a website—all of those questions can be debated freely. Suffice it to say we went through numerous iterations to arrive at the label we are proposing. We put it out here not as an end but as a beginning.

Every packaged food label would feature a color-coded bar with a 15-point scale so that almost instantly the consumer could determine whether the product's overall rating fell between 11 and 15 (green), 6 and 10 (yellow), or 0 and 5 (red). This alone could be enough for a fair snap decision. (We've also got a box to indicate the presence or absence of GMOs.)

We arrive at the score by rating three key factors, each of which comprises numerous subfactors. The first is the obvious "Nutrition," about which little needs to be said. High sugar, trans fats, the presence of micronutrients and fiber, and so on would all be taken into account. Thus soda would rate a zero and frozen broccoli might rate a five. (It's hard to imagine labeling fresh vegetables.)

The second is "Foodness." This assesses just how close the product is to real food. White bread made with bleached flour, yeast conditioners, and preservatives would get a zero or one; so would soda; a candy bar high in sugar but made with real ingredients would presumably score low on nutrition but could get a higher score on "foodness"; here, frozen broccoli would rate a four.

The third is the broadest (and trickiest); we're calling it "Welfare." This would include the treatment of workers, animals, and the earth. Are workers treated like animals? Are animals produced like widgets? Is environmental damage significant? If the answer to those three questions is "yes"—as it might be, for example, with industrially produced chickens—then the score would be zero, or close to it. If the labor force is treated fairly and animals well, and waste is insignificant or recycled, the score would be higher.

These are not simple calculations, but neither can one honestly say that they're impossible to perform. It may well be that there are wiser ways to sort through this information and get it across. The main point here is: let's get started.

OCTOBER 13, 2012

Rethinking the Word "Foodie"

A t a dinner party the other night where people were asked to say a word about themselves, one woman said, "My name is"—whatever it was—"and I'm a foodie." I cringed.

I'm not proud of that visceral reaction; in fact, I think it's wrong. But I do wish there were a stronger, less demeaning-sounding word than "foodie" for someone who cares about good food, but as seems so often the case, there is not. Witness the near-meaningless-ness of "natural" and "vegetarian" and the inadequacy of "organic" and "vegan." But proposing new words is a fool's game; rather, let's try to make the word "foodie" a tad more meaningful.

As it stands, many self-described foodies are new-style epicures. And there's nothing destructive about watching competitive cooking shows, doing "anything" to get a table at the trendy restaurant, scouring the web for single-estate farro, or devoting oneself to finding the best food truck. The problem arises when it stops there.

More conscious foodies understand that producing food has an effect beyond creating an opportunity for pleasure. And this woman was not atypical: She's into sustainability ("We have to grow our food better, right?"), organic (though for all I know this means organic junk food), and local food. She shops at farmers' markets when she can. She cooks.

We can't ask everyone who likes eating—which, given enough time and an adequate income, includes everyone I've ever met—to become a food activist. But to increase the consciousness levels of well-intentioned foodies, it might be useful to sketch out what "caring about good food" means, and to try to move "foodie" to a place where it refers to someone who gets beyond fun to pay attention to how food is produced and the impact it has.

The qualities that characterize good food vary within a narrow range. Good food is real, it's healthy, it's produced sustainably, it's fair, and it's affordable. Maybe it's prepared at home, though if communal kitchens or restaurants can deliver those qualities, I'm all for that.

None of this is complicated, but simple doesn't mean easy. "Real" means traditional; if it existed 100 years ago, it's probably real. Hyperprocessed is neither real nor healthy. No single factor is causing our diet-related health crisis, but some things we eat are making us sick and it's more likely that the culprits are added sugars, not asparagus. So, "healthy" most likely will always be "whole" or even "real." This doesn't mean we should eat more watercress because it's a superfood, high in some supposedly critical nutrient, but it does mean we want to eat more fruits and vegetables. As we know.

"Sustainable" (or "green," another word that's been rendered near-meaningless) suggests resource-neutral, or as close to it as we can come. There is farming, not necessarily organic, that puts as much back into the soil as it extracts; it also uses water in a way that will guarantee a supply for the future. We can call that "sustainable."

"Fair" and "affordable" are very tough. As Margaret Gray discusses in her excellent book, *Labor and the Locavore*, we cannot achieve ethical consistency in producing food without paying attention to labor. (Animals are important too, but I suppose I'm an anthro-chauvinist.) For food to be affordable, people—all people—must earn living wages; alternatively, good food must be subsidized. Both conditions would be even better. (As almost every foodie knows, we're currently subsidizing bad food.)

Some of these qualities can be controlled by individuals: Most of us can eat real and healthier food easily enough, and, as it happens, growing such food tends to be more sustainable. On a grand scale, we need societal changes and government support to make this more accessible to everyone. But—and this is the part I like best—making good food fair and affordable cannot be achieved without affecting the whole system. These are not just food questions; they are questions of justice and equality and rights, of enhancing rather than restricting democracy, of making a more rational, legitimate economy. In other words, working to make food fair and affordable is an opportunity for this country to live up to its founding principles.

So shifting the implications of "foodie" means shifting our culture to one in which eaters—that's everyone—realize that buying into the current food "system" means exploiting animals, people, and the environment, and making ourselves sick. To change that, we have to change not only the way we behave as individuals but the way we behave as a society. It's rewarding to find the best pork bun; it's even more rewarding to fight for a good food system at the same time. That's what we foodies do.

JUNE 24, 2014

Hunger in Plain Sight

There are hungry people out there, actually; they're just largely invisible to the rest of us, or they look so much like us that it's hard to tell. The Supplemental Assistance Nutrition Program, better known as SNAP and even better known as food stamps, currently has around 46 million participants, a record high. That's one in eight Americans—10 people in your subway car, one or two on every line at Walmart.

We wouldn't wish that on anyone, but as it stands, the number should: many people are unaware that they're eligible for SNAP, and thus the participation rate is probably around three-quarters of what it should be.

Food stamps allow you to shop more or less normally, but on an extremely tight budget, around $130 a month. It's tough to feed a family on food stamps (and even tougher without them), and that's where food banks—a network of nonprofit, nongovernment agencies, centrally located clearinghouses for donated or purchased food that is sent to local affiliated agencies or "pantries"— come in. Food banks may cover an entire state or part of one: the Regional Food Bank of Oklahoma, for example, serves 53 counties and provides enough food to feed 48,000 square miles and feeds 90,000 people a week—in a state with fewer than four million people.

Like many other food banks, Oklahoma's, says executive director Rodney, has made a commitment to serve every single person in need in its area; put that together with that state's geography, and it might give you pause. Similarly, God's Love We Deliver (not technically a food bank), which provides over a million cooked meals a year to sick people in the five boroughs and the Newark area, has seen its numbers nearly double in the last six years because, as Karen

Pearl, the president and C.E.O. told me, "We are never going to have a waiting list and are never going to turn people away."

And because poverty is growing.

Lyndon Johnson's Great Society programs brought the poverty level down to 11 percent from 20 percent in less than 10 years. Ronald Reagan began the process of dismantling that minimal safety net, and as a result the current poverty level is close to 16 percent, and food stamps are not fully doing their job. "There was a time in this country," says Maryland Food Bank president and C.E.O. Deborah Flateman, "when food stamps had practically eliminated hunger; then the big cuts happened, and we've been trying to recover ever since."

Food banks are changing. During a visit to the Rhode Island Community Food Bank I was surprised to see not rows and rows of mac 'n' cheese and Frosted Flakes but fresh produce, rice and beans, even meat. That's because until recently, manufacturers' mistakes—the misprinted label, the too-soon sell-by date—went to food banks; now there are fewer mistakes, and "seconds" are usually sold to "dollar" stores rather than donated.

In addition, the cutbacks to The Emergency Food Assistance Program (Tefap), a Department of Agriculture program that delivers purchased food to states for free distribution—usually through food banks—have hit hard; in Oklahoma, for example, the food bank lost around six million pounds of donated food from Tefap, representing something like 70 percent. (At the same time, Bivens notes, apples went from $14 to $24 a case.)

These developments cause hardships, but opportunities too: every food bank I spoke with is providing its clients with more fresh produce and real food than before. (And less junk: Andrew Schiff, who runs the Rhode Island Community Food Bank, convinced his board years ago that they did not need to give people free soda. "We provide meals," he told me, and "soda and chips does not constitute a meal.")

Food banks closest to where food is grown in quantity are in the best shape to obtain produce. The San Francisco and Marin Food Banks, according to executive director Paul Ash, get "10 or 15 truckloads of produce a week out of growing areas like California's Central Valley," some of which it shares with food banks as far away as upstate New York. Nor is this solely a West Coast phenomenon: the Maryland Food Bank, says Flateman, went from working with two farms two years ago to 51 in 2012.

This all sounds great: providing people in need with real food is clearly preferable to providing them with junk. But, as Ash says, only one out of two people who are eligible for SNAP in his state are on the program, and "the only thing that can really touch that problem would be improving SNAP, because there aren't enough warehouses in San Francisco for organizations like ours to take up that slack." Ideally, SNAP would work so well that food banks became superfluous.

Furthermore, as great as fresh produce is, the reality is that most people need more than onions, carrots, apples, and oranges. And so it's dried goods like rice and beans and concentrated protein like animal products that cost food banks real money. And there are other issues: you don't have to know how to cook to "prepare" cold cereal, or even boxed mac 'n' cheese. But "people don't know how to prepare rice and beans anymore," says Bivens, who along with others I spoke to is doing two things: increasingly preparing cooked, shelf-stable food to give to people and offering cooking lessons.

SNAP participants and food bank visitors are sometimes homeless people but they're also our neighbors, our employees, our co-workers, our fellow bus riders, the family in the car next to ours, the cashier at the supermarket; more and more, they're our parents, because Social Security is another program that isn't cutting it.

The need is everywhere. Whether you look at this from a moral perspective (love thy neighbor, remember?) or a practical one, it's clear that SNAP and food banks deserve better funding, not worse.

It seems absurd to have to say it, but no one in this country should go hungry.

NOVEMBER 27, 2012

Can Big Food Regulate Itself?
Fat Chance

L ife would be so much easier if we could only set our own guidelines. You could define the average weight as 10 pounds higher than your own and, voilà, no more obesity! You could raise the speed limit to 90 miles per hour and never worry about a ticket. You could call a cholesterol level of 250 "normal" and celebrate with a bag of fried pork rinds. (You could even claim that cutting government spending would increase employment, but that might be going too far.) You could certainly turn junk food into something "healthy."

That's what the food industry is doing.

In May of 2011 I wrote about the voluntary guidelines for marketing junk food to kids developed by an interagency group headed by the Federal Trade Commission. These nonbinding suggestions ask that the industry market real food to kids instead of the junk they so famously favor selling. But the industry argues that the recommendations are effectively mandatory because noncompliance would lead to retaliation and eliminate all food advertising to adolescents, as well as 74,000 jobs.

On the phone last week, Representative Rosa DeLauro, a Democrat from Connecticut, told me that even though the guidelines are "without teeth," the pushback from the industry has been formidable: "We have seen political showmanship, misinformation about the impact of these voluntary guidelines, insistence that the industry has been successful in self-regulation and that these efforts would violate the First Amendment."

That voluntary guidelines could curb the right to free speech is absurd, but not as wacky as letting the industry set its own standards. Yet that's what has happened: The Children's Food and Beverage Advertising Initiative (CFBAI), a group of food manufacturers that includes McDonald's, Burger King, PepsiCo, and Kraft Foods, came up with its own guidelines defining foods healthy enough to market to kids. (It's worth mentioning another group, too—if just to admire its name, The Sensible Food Policy Coalition—led by PepsiCo, Kellogg's, General Mills, and other big companies, evidently created solely to prevent the voluntary guidelines from gaining a foothold.)

CFBAI is a champion of "self-regulation," which means repeating a series of mantras that include "facts" like "there is no such thing as good food and bad food," or that Cookie Crisp cereal (or dozens of others) "can be a part of a balanced diet," all the while micro-adjusting hyperprocessed food so that "more fiber" and "less sugar" aren't outright lies, even though the food itself can hardly be claimed to be "less junky." With self-regulation, even Singles can be considered "part of a balanced diet."

And guess what? In general, the companies fare well in meeting their own standards (which, pathetically, the F.T.C. sees as a "significant advance"): two-thirds of the products they advertise are A-O.K., with the remainder requiring just modest adjustments. See? Mission accomplished! Corn Pops are now healthy!

Another example: last week, McDonald's promised a minor tweak of its Happy Meal (which, of course, "can be part of a well-balanced diet for kids"), adding a few apple slices, removing a few French fries, and making milk—chocolate or regular—a more prominent option. It still comes with a toy, and soda will remain a choice. (I'm not sure anyone is claiming soda is part of a healthy diet, but stay tuned.) The move received widespread praise, with Michelle Obama leading the cheers.

But despite the seal of approval of our first lady/self-appointed nutrition expert, a Happy Meal with a piece of apple is still a box of branded, overpriced junk food sold not by its value but by its marketing scheme. (Forty percent of McDonald's advertising budget is spent on marketing to kids.)

This is not "progress," but a public relations victory along with—as Michele Simon points out in her blog—an attempt to short-circuit regulations and laws that have some guts, like the one in San Francisco that forbids the inclusion of toys in meals that don't meet reasonable nutrition standards. The last thing McDonald's or any like corporation wants to see is a strong, activist government protecting consumers, whether or not they're capable of adult judgment or are habituated (a harsher word is "addicted") to self-destructive products.

Self-regulation may be immediate, nonthreatening, and magical, but it doesn't work. A study published in the *Archives of Pediatrics and Adolescent Medicine* by Dr. Lisa Powell and other researchers at the University of Illinois at Chicago tracked changes in exposure for all food, beverage, and restaurant TV ads seen by kids from 2 to 11 years old, from 2003 to 2009. It found that, overall, daily exposure to the ads declined but the percentage among companies that had pledged to self-regulate was higher than those that didn't. And in 2009, 86 percent of these ads still featured unhealthy foods.

What's worse? Self-serving self-regulation or toothless guidelines set by an agency that appears to be complicit in maintaining the status quo? Hard to say. What's better is having grassroots movements that drive agencies toward real regulation.

AUGUST 2, 2011

Tobacco, Firearms, and Food

Let's say your beliefs include the notion that hard work will bring good things to you, that the golden rule is a nice idea though it may occasionally have limits, and that it's more or less every person for him- or herself. Your overall guiding force is not altruism, but you're not immoral; you're a good citizen, and you don't break any major laws. This could describe many of us; most, maybe.

Now suppose you're in the business of producing, marketing, or selling tobacco or firearms—products known to sometimes kill others. You need not be a corporate executive or a criminal arms dealer; you might be a retailer of cigarettes, a person who sells them along with magazines, a marketer, a gun shop owner. In any case, your conscience is clear: you're selling regulated legal products and, as long as you're obeying the regulations, you're doing nothing illegal. ("Wrong" is a judgment call.)

You sleep well, believing that the government would further regulate your product if it were necessary. And if regulations were to change, you'd change with them. But to act otherwise—to hold back your energy from production or sales just because of moral or social pressure—would be foolish, and put you at a competitive disadvantage.

For many years after knowing about the lethal nature of tobacco, our government did little or nothing to limit its consumption. That's changed gradually in the last 50 years, and more dramatically since 1998, because of successful lawsuits and because the Food and Drug Administration often tries to pursue its mission. (For a variety of reasons not worth going into, firearms are more challenging to regulate. Let's leave it at that for now.)

O.K., so suppose we pass legislation that discourages you from producing or selling tobacco or firearms while at the same time actively encouraging you—supporting you—to change to producing apples or cotton or washing machines or screwdrivers; as long as you could see a way to increase profit, you'd probably look at the new opportunity. After all, it's not as if you want to produce agents of death. You want to make the best living you can selling stuff that's legal and that people want. Markets change, and flexibility is important, and the government can and does affect your business, even if it's by inaction.

Now let's apply this same way of thinking to the major food categories—and for the purposes of this discussion there are only three—and what it's like to be a farmer or producer, or a manufacturer, processor, distributor, retailer of this stuff. Again, you're agnostic about what you sell, but you're profit-conscious. And the government can and does affect your business; it can help your business ("you didn't build it yourself") or hurt it, as it should if your business is harming others.

Let's call the first food group industrially produced animal products. Producing and selling as much as possible is the way to go here, since the penalties for damage your product does to human and animal health and to the environment (including climate) are virtually nonexistent. You can treat the animals as you like and damn the consequences, from salmonella contamination to antibiotic resistance to water contamination to, of course, cruelty. There are even incentives, in the form of subsidized prices for animal feed.

The next group is most easily labeled junk food; you might call it "hyperprocessed." This comprises aisles and aisles of "edibles" sold in supermarkets and restaurants, and is often "food" that's unrecognizable as such, ranging from soda and other sugar-sweetened beverages to things like chicken nuggets and Pringles and tens of thousands of other examples. These are mostly made from commodity crops, especially corn, soybeans, and wheat. Federal subsidies abound in many forms here, from direct payments (in theory, these are ending, to be replaced by a bizarre form of crop insurance) to the ethanol mandate to virtually unregulated land use that permits toxic overapplication of fertilizers and other chemicals. There is also that same failure to recognize the public health and environmental costs of what is probably the least healthy diet a wealthy nation could devise. You could even say that the Supplemental Nutrition Assistance Program (SNAP, usually called food stamps) acts as a subsidy to junk food, since nothing limits using food stamps for food that promotes disease. It's worth noting that for the past century the bulk of university research, much of it paid for with tax dollars, has gone into figuring out how to increase the yield of the crops and processes that turn out this junk that sickens.

Then, in the third group, there's everything else, from fruits and vegetables—absurdly called "specialty crops" by the Department of Agriculture—to animals raised in sustainable and even humane ways. But here, disincentives abound: farmers may be encouraged to allow some land to go fallow, but not to be planted in specialty crops, and research money, subsidies, insurance, market promotion, and access to credit are directed toward industrial food production, distribution, and sales. These inefficiencies make most of this real food, which is health-promoting and closer to environmentally neutral, appear to be more expensive. (Only "appear," though. If you account for the costs of environmental and public health damage, industrially produced junk food and animal products actually cost more.)

In a neutral ("free") market, there'd be more room for producers and processors of fruits and vegetables to make money by responding to increased demand for wholesome fruits and vegetables without competing with subsidized junk food. In a sane—let's say properly regulated—market, there'd be incentives for agriculture that benefited both grower and consumer with products that were less damaging to the environment and public health. Food stamps, for example, would be restricted to use for nourishing food. Direct subsidies might be used to encourage new farmers who wanted to grow "specialty crops" rather than for farmers working thousands of acres of corn.

One could imagine a government that encourages more life-giving (and less disease-causing) agriculture just as one can acknowledge that sanity prevails when government steeply taxes tobacco and encourages its farmers to move on to something else. (I'm not saying, by the way, that tobacco farmers have been treated fairly; much more could have been done—and still could be done—to help them transition to other profitable crops.)

Of course this is disruptive; change the status quo, and someone is hurt. But the public health disaster created by our commodity-pushing agricultural policies is only getting worse, and calls for the same kind of action in industrial agriculture that we've seen in tobacco and, to a lesser extent, in guns. That kind of action will happen only when we have political representatives who care about food, health, and the environment.

We can pressure corporations all we want, and what we'll get, mostly, is healthier junk food. Really, though, as long as sugar is profitable and

100 percent unrestricted (and subsidized and protected!), marketers will try to get 2-year-olds hooked on soda and Gatorade.

But the job of government is not to encourage profitable businesses at the cost of public health; it's to regulate them so that the public is served.

JANUARY 14, 2014

Don't End Agricultural Subsidies, Fix Them

Agricultural subsidies have helped bring us high-fructose corn syrup, factory farming, fast food, a two-soda-a-day habit and its accompanying obesity, the near-demise of family farms, monoculture, and a host of other ills.

Yet—like so many government programs—what subsidies need is not the ax, but reform that moves them forward. Imagine support designed to encourage a resurgence of small- and medium-size farms producing not corn syrup and animal feed but food we can touch, see, buy, and eat—like apples and carrots—while diminishing handouts to agribusiness and its political cronies.

Farm subsidies were created in an attempt to ameliorate the effects of the Great Depression, which makes it ironic that in an era when more Americans are suffering financially than at any time since, these subsidies are mostly going to those who need them least.

That wasn't the plan, of course. In the 1930s, prices were fixed on a variety of commodities, and some farmers were paid to reduce their crop yields. The program was supported by a tax on processors of food—now there's a precedent!—and was intended to be temporary. It worked, sort of: prices rose and more farmers survived. But land became concentrated in the hands of fewer farmers, and agribusiness was born, and along with it the sad joke that the government paid farmers for not growing crops.

The Farm Bill, up for renewal in 2012, includes an agricultural subsidy portion worth up to $30 billion, $5 billion of which is what you might call handouts, direct payments to farmers.

The subsidy-suckers don't grow the fresh fruits and vegetables that should be dominating our diet. Indeed, if all Americans decided to actually eat the five servings a day of fruits and vegetables that are recommended, they would discover that American agriculture isn't set up to meet that need. They grow what they're paid to grow: corn, soy, wheat, cotton, and rice.

The first two of these are the pillars for the typical American diet—featuring an unnaturally large consumption of meat, never-before-seen junk food, and a bizarre avoidance of plants—as well as the fortunes of Pepsi, Dunkin' Donuts, KFC, and the others that have relied on cheap corn and soy to build their empires of unhealthful food. Over the years, prices of fresh produce have risen, while those of meat, poultry, sweets, fats, and oils, and especially soda, have fallen. (Tom Philpott, writing in the environment and food website Grist and citing a Tufts University study, reckons that between 1997 and 2005 subsidies saved chicken, pork, beef, and HFCS producers roughly $26.5 billion. In the short term, that saved consumers money too—prices for these foods are unjustifiably low—but at what cost to the environment, our food choices, and our health?)

Eliminating the $5 billion in direct agricultural payments would level the playing field for farmers who grow nonsubsidized crops, but just a bit—perhaps not even noticeably. There would probably be a decrease in the amount of HFCS in the market, in the 10 billion animals we "process" annually, in the ethanol used to fill gas-guzzlers, and in the soy from which we chemically extract oil for frying potatoes and chicken. Those are all benefits, which we could compound by taking those billions and using them for things like high-speed rail, fulfilling our promises to public workers, maintaining Pell grants for low-income college students, or any other number of worthy, forward-thinking causes.

But let's not kid ourselves. Although the rage for across-the-board spending cuts doesn't extend to the public—according to a recent Pew poll, most people want no cuts or even increased spending in major areas—once the $5 billion is gone, it's not coming back.

That the current system is a joke is barely arguable: wealthy growers are paid even in good years, and may receive drought aid when there's no drought. It's become so bizarre that some homeowners lucky enough to have bought land that once grew rice now have subsidized lawns. Fortunes have been paid to Fortune 500 companies and even gentlemen farmers like David Rockefeller.

Thus even House Speaker Boehner calls the bill a "slush fund"; the powerful Iowa Farm Bureau suggests that direct payments end; and Glenn Beck is on the bandwagon. (This last should make you suspicious.) Not surprisingly, many Tea Partiers happily accept subsidies, including Vicky Hartzler (R-MO, $775,000), Stephen Fincher (R-TN, $2.5 million), and Michele Bachmann (R-MN, $250,000). No hypocrisy there.

Left and right can perhaps agree that these are payments we don't need to make. But suppose we use this money to steer our agriculture—and our health—in the right direction. A Gallup poll indicates that most Americans oppose cutting aid to farmers, and presumably they're not including David Rockefeller or Michele Bachmann in that protected group; we still think of farmers as stewards of the land, and the closer that sentiment is to reality the better off we'll be.

By making the program more sensible the money could benefit us all. For example, it could:

- Fund research and innovation in sustainable agriculture, so that in the long run we can get the system on track.

- Provide necessary incentives to attract the 100,000 new farmers Secretary of Agriculture Vilsack claims we need.

- Save more farmland from development.

- Provide support for farmers who grow currently unsubsidized fruits, vegetables, and beans, while providing incentives for monoculture commodity farmers to convert some of their operations to these more desirable foods.

- Level the playing field so that medium-sized farms—big enough to supply local supermarkets but small enough to care what and how they grow—can become more competitive with agribusiness.

The point is that this money, which is already in the budget, could encourage the development of the kind of agriculture we need, one that prioritizes caring for the land, the people who work it, and the people who need the real food that's grown on it.

We could, of course, finance or even augment the program with new monies, by taking a clue from the '30s, when the farm subsidy program began: Let the food giants that have profited so mightily and long from cheap corn and soy—that have not so far been asked to share the pain—pay for it.

MARCH 2, 2011

Stop Subsidizing Obesity

Not long ago few doctors—not even pediatricians—concerned themselves much with nutrition. This has changed, and dramatically: As childhood obesity gains recognition as a true health crisis, more and more doctors are publicly expressing alarm at the impact the standard American diet is having on health.

"I never saw Type 2 diabetes during my training, 20 years ago," David Ludwig, a pediatrician, told me the other day, referring to what was once called "adult-onset" diabetes, the form that is often caused by obesity. "Never. Now about a quarter of the new diabetes cases we're seeing are Type 2."

Ludwig, who is director of the New Balance Foundation Obesity Prevention Center in Boston, is one of three authors, all medical doctors, of an essay ("Viewpoint") in the *Journal of the American Medical Association* titled "Opportunities to Reduce Childhood Hunger and Obesity."

That title that would once have been impossible, but now it's merely paradoxical. Because the situation is this: 17 percent of children in the United States are obese, 16 percent are food-insecure (this means they have inconsistent access to food), and some number, which is impossible to nail down, are both. Seven times as many poor children are obese as those who are underweight, an indication that government aid in the form of food stamps, now officially called SNAP, does a good job of addressing hunger but encourages the consumption of unhealthy calories.

The doctors' piece, which addresses these issues, was written by Ludwig along with Susan Blumenthal, a former assistant Surgeon General and U.S.D.A. medical adviser, and Walter Willett, chair of Harvard's Department of Nutrition (and a stalwart of sound nutrition research for more than 30 years). It's essentially a plea to tweak SNAP regulations (Supplemental Nutrition Assistance Benefits, the program formerly and more familiarly known as food stamps) so that the program concerns itself with the quality of calories instead of just their quantity.

"It's shocking," says Ludwig, "how little we consider food quality in the management of chronic diseases. And in the case of SNAP that failure costs taxpayers twice: We pay once when low-income families buy junk foods and sugary beverages with SNAP benefits, and we pay a second time when poor diet quality inevitably increases the costs of health care in general, and Medicaid and Medicare in particular."

The argument that soda and other junk masquerading as food should be made ineligible for purchase by food stamps, as are alcohol and tobacco, is one that's been gaining momentum in the last few years. It's also one that has led to a split in what might be called the nutrition advocacy community.

On the one side are "anti-hunger" groups who want to maintain SNAP's status quo; on the other are those who believe SNAP must be protected but also that it must be adjusted to take into account the changes in agriculture, marketing, and diet that have occurred since SNAP was born 50 years ago, changes that have led to the obesity crisis.

I'm in that second camp, as are the authors of this article, who make a case that the rift is artificial, though both sides share the same fear: if we advocate any tinkering with SNAP, it may make the program more vulnerable to cuts that it can ill afford.

But the reality is that some billions of SNAP dollars (exact figures are unavailable, but the number most experts use is four) are being spent on soda, which is strictly speaking not food, and certainly not a nutritious substance, and is a leading cause of obesity. Seven percent of our calories come from sugar-sweetened beverages, none of them doing any of us any good.

Though there were those who argued against including soda when food stamps were created, the most pressing need was to address calorie deficiency, and that remains important. But the situation is different now: we recognize the harmful properties of added sugar, the importance of high-quality nutrients in children has been better analyzed, and obesity is a bigger problem than hunger. So funding low-quality, harmful calories is detrimental to both funders and recipients.

"It's time," says Ludwig, "for us to realize that the goals of anti-hunger and obesity prevention are not at cross purposes. In fact, poor-quality foods can actually increase hunger because they are inherently less filling." A child will become hungrier, sooner, after consuming 200 calories from a sugary beverage, compared to an apple and peanut butter with the same calories.

What's to be done? How to improve the quality of calories purchased by SNAP recipients? The answer is easy: Make sure that SNAP dollars are spent on nutritious food.

This could happen in two ways: first, remove the subsidy for sugar-sweetened beverages, since no one without a share in the profits can argue that the substance plays a constructive role in any diet. "There's no rationale for continuing to subsidize them through SNAP benefits," says Ludwig, "with the level of science we have linking their consumption to obesity, diabetes, and heart disease." New York City proposed a pilot program that would do precisely this back in 2011; it was rejected by the Department of Agriculture (U.S.D.A.) as "too complex."

Simultaneously, make it easier to buy real food; several cities, including New York, have programs that double the value of food stamps when used for purchases at farmers' markets. The next step is to similarly increase the spending power of food stamps when they're used to buy fruits, vegetables, legumes, and whole grains, not just in farmers' markets but in supermarkets—indeed, everywhere people buy food.

Both of these could be set up as pilot programs by the U.S.D.A. (The department already finances a similar pilot program—known as the Health Incentives Pilot—in Hampden County, Mass., but it is tiny and is scheduled to end soon.) Their inevitable success would lead to their expansion, and ultimately to better health for SNAP participants, who now number nearly 50 million. The impact of improving the diet of that many Americans would be profound; the impact of not doing so is tragic.

DECEMBER 25, 2012

Fixing Our Food Problem

Nothing affects public health in the United States more than food. Gun violence kills tens of thousands of Americans a year. Heart disease, cancer, stroke, and diabetes kill more than a million people a year—nearly half of all deaths—and diet is a root cause of many of those diseases.

And the root of that dangerous diet is our system of hyper-industrial agriculture, the kind that uses 10 times as much energy as it produces.

We must figure out a way to un-invent this food system. It's been a major contributor to climate change, spawned the obesity crisis, poisoned countless volumes of land and water, wasted energy, tortured billions of animals ... I could go on. The point is that "sustainability" is not only possible but essential: only by saving the earth can we save ourselves, and vice versa.

How do we do that?

This seems like a good day to step back a bit and suggest something that's sometimes difficult to accept.

Patience.

We can only dismantle this system little by little, and slowly. Change takes time. Often—usually—that time exceeds the life span of its pioneers. And when it comes to sustainable food for billions, we're the pioneers of a food movement that's just beginning to take shape. The abolition movement began at least a century before the Civil War, 200 years before the civil rights movement. The struggle to gain the right to vote for women in the United States was active for 75 years before an amendment was passed. The gay rights struggle has made tremendous strides over the last 40 years, but equal treatment under the law is hardly established.

Activists who took on these issues had in common a clear series of demands and a sense that the work was ongoing. They had a large and ever-growing public following and a willingness to sacrifice time, energy, and even life for the benefit not only of contemporaries but for subsequent generations.

They were also aware that there is no success without a willingness to fail; that failure is a part of progress. A single defeat was seen as a temporary setback. The same vision should be applied to every issue the nascent food movement is tackling.

Yet before we can assess our progress, we must state our goals. There is no consensus behind a program for achieving sustainable production of food that promotes rather than attacks health. We can't ask for "better food for all"; we must be specific. In the very near term, for example, we must fight to protect and improve programs that make food available to lower-income Americans. We must also support the increasingly assertive battles of workers in food-related industries; nothing reflects our moral core more accurately than the abuses we overlook in the names of convenience and economy.

Beyond that, I believe that the two issues that will have the greatest reverberations in agriculture, health, and the environment are reducing the consumption of sugar-laden beverages and improving the living conditions of livestock.

About the first I have written plenty, and can summarize: when we begin treating sugar-sweetened beverages as we do tobacco, we will make a huge stride in improving our diet.

The second is even more powerful, and progress was made in that arena in 2012 as one food company after another resolved to (eventually) reject pork produced with gestation crates. So over the next few years, some animals will be treated somewhat better. This is absolutely, unquestionably thanks to public pressure, which should now set its sights higher and insist that all animals grown for food production be treated not just better but well.

Well-cared-for animals will necessarily be more expensive, which means we'll eat fewer of them; that's a win-win. They'll use fewer antibiotics, they'll be produced by more farmers in more places, and they'll eat less commodity grain, which will both reduce environmental damage and allow for more land to be used for high-quality human food like fruits and vegetables.

Allies may argue that I miss the mark with either or both of these, and that's fine: it's a discussion. The point is that no major food issue will be resolved in the next 10 years. As pioneers, we must build upon incremental progress and not be disheartened, because often there isn't quick resolution for complex issues.

An association between tobacco and cancer was discovered more than 200 years ago. The surgeon general's report that identified smoking as a public health issue appeared in 1964. The food movement has not yet reached its 1964; there isn't even a general acknowledgment of a problem in need of fixing.

So, let's call for energy, action—and patience.

JANUARY 1, 2013

A Few Final Thoughts

Why Take Food Seriously?

Our relationship with food is changing more rapidly than ever, and like many others, I've watched in awe. As a food journalist and author for 30 years, my perspective has been unusual: I've worked with influential people in the field while remaining in frequent contact with my readers, who are some unknowable percentage of the home-cooking, food-obsessed segment of the public.

I've never been more hopeful. (In fact, I was never hopeful at all until recently.) Each year, each month it sometimes seems, there are more signs that convenience, that mid-20th-century curse word, may give way to quality—even what you might call wholesomeness—just before we all turn into the shake-sucking fatties of *Wall-E*.

We are taking food seriously again.

Until 50 years ago, of course, every household had at least one person who took food seriously every day. But from the 1950s on, the majority of the population began contentedly cooking less and less, eating out more and more, and devouring food that was worse and worse, until the horrible global slop served by fast-food and "casual dining" chains came to dominate the scene. One result: an unprecedented rise in obesity levels and a not-unrelated climb in health care costs.

Yet we would not let food go to hell permanently, at least not without a fight. And even at its nadir there were signs of awakening. Beginning in the 1960s, more Americans than ever discovered France, Italy, Mexico, Japan, and other countries, where traditional cooking remained intact. Revised immigration laws gave us a new and varied influx of immigrants, whose previously rare cuisines—Tibetan, Cambodian, Ethiopian, and Ecuadorean, for example—

became visible in many cities. At the same time, people like Julia Child, Marcella Hazan, and Julie Sahni made once-exotic cuisines accessible for amateurs.

Nevertheless many Americans began applying the word "cooking" to the act of defrosting and heating mass-produced frozen food in a microwave oven. Still, by the mid-'80s there were new vistas for food lovers. There was a nascent food-as-art scene, presaging Ferran Adrià. Old-style French food—the fancy stuff, with sauces—died a quick death (thank you, Paul Bocuse). Fantastic local ingredients, treated minimally, became all the rage (thank you, Alice Waters and friends). European chefs in the United States embraced Asian ingredients (thank you, Jean-Georges Vongerichten).

At first these changes affected few people. But a confluence of factors—new cuisines, a cultural fixation on health, frustration with low-quality food—led to a renewed appreciation of eating and home cooking. Logically, this led to an increased awareness of industrially raised animals and overprocessed food and ultimately to an interest in local ingredients, in vegetables, in sustainability, in human health.

Then there was food television. We were ripe for the Food Network's Emeril, Rachael, Mario, and Bobby, who created a buzz based on celebrity that grabbed not only the middle-aged and the young but also the very young. And when 6-year-olds started wanting to be chefs—that was different.

The news wasn't all good. At the millennium, we knew that fish had disappeared from the seas, taste had disappeared from chickens, regulation had all but disappeared from government agencies, and humanity had disappeared from the way we handle animals. Obesity and its associated lifestyle diseases became news, as did acute illnesses like salmonella and mad cow. It also became clear to everyone who took the time to think that our overconsumption of meat was contributing to the hunger of nearly one billion fellow earthlings.

This has led many Americans to think as much about food as they do about *Survivor* or the N.F.L.—which is to say a lot—and its preparation is no longer limited to what was once called a housewife. The unrelenting pressure on women to join the workforce encouraged (forced?) men to at least learn how to turn on the stove; from there, many of them took to cooking enthusiastically (some, no doubt, because so many gadgets are involved). Those children who dream of being chefs share in the cooking; nearly every young person I meet cooks routinely.

Of course, food continues to be fetishized; organic food has been commodified; the federal government subsidizes almost all of the wrong kinds of food production; supermarkets peddle way too much nonreal food ("junk food" or, to use my mother's word, "dreck"); and weight-loss diets still discourage common-sense eating. But questions like "Would you prefer a mass-produced organic grape from Chile or a nonorganic one from a backyard vine in Upstate New York?" are more common in conversation, and the dialogue about food routinely includes words like locavore, vegetarian, sustainable, and flexitarian.

The real issues—how do we grow and raise, distribute and sell, prepare and eat food? And how do our patterns of doing these things affect the rest of the world (and vice versa)?—are simply too big to ignore.

And if we are obsessing about where our food is from and how it's grown rather than whether our fries are cooked in beef fat or "cholesterol-free oil" (or, even worse, whether our gold-leaf-topped foie gras is good for us), this is progress.

Simply put, many more Americans are seeing food as more than a necessary fuel whose only requirement is that it can be obtained and consumed without much difficulty or cost. Perhaps just in time, we're saying, "Hold the shake," and looking for something more wholesome.

OCTOBER 12, 2008

Do Sweat the Small Stuff

My life is a strange dichotomy. In between writing these columns, and my books, and the other activities I'm involved in that tend to be semi-solitary pursuits, I spend my time traveling back and forth across the country promoting those same undertakings. Which means I routinely find myself in a room full of people asking some questions that I'll never be able to answer and others that I can, confidently.

A thoughtful answer to a single question is usually about the length of a paragraph in this column. Longer answers would limit the interviewer and members of the audience of their chance to voice their concerns. So in a way, the more difficult the question, the shorter the answer. For example:

"How do we change the food system?"

A: Slowly. One step at a time.

"How do you define 'real food'"?

A: It existed 100 years ago.

"What do you think about GMOs?"

A: Both fear and benefits are overrated.

"What are the biggest problems in food?"

A: Unregulated junk, unregulated marketing, barely regulated antibiotics.

"What about people who can't afford real food, or don't have access to fresh produce or kitchens that are safe and equipped for cooking?"

A: These are justice issues, not food issues. Of course they're important, but they also serve to point out that when you address food issues seriously, you must also address broader, systemic issues like those of inequality.

"What can I do to help change things in the food world?"

A: If you care about real food, and you keep caring about it, it almost doesn't matter what your job is; you'll help make real change.

These are common questions from both interviewers and the public. But when people approach me individually, the questions change. One on one is more personal and feels more meaningful.

They're questions I've answered a thousand times: What do I do with chard? Should I buy organic food? When and how should I salt pasta water? How do I feed my kids? What do you eat when you have nothing in the house? How can I eat a decent lunch? How important is local food? What do you do with turnips?

The questions show how important food really is to people, even though they may appear trivial. They're easier, but they're meaningful, because their answers are empowering rather than frustrating.

And this is what I try to emphasize: We can look at the big issues, we should look at the big issues, but the big issues can be discouraging. We've made a little progress, and I'm confident we'll make much more, but changing the food system is a big battle, a war even, and winning it will take campaign finance reform and a more representative House and perhaps even the abolition of the Senate as well as a whole lot of restructuring and re-regulating.

When we talk about changing the food system, we talk about changing just about everything. So we should be prepared for sudden change—it could happen (see: gay marriage)—but we should expect a long and difficult struggle. We won't, in the near future, see a ban on marketing junk food to children—perhaps as important a childhood issue as there is right now—any sooner than we'll see the national minimum wage raised to $15.

So much of this is so big that it's out of our individual control, and it's easy to become disheartened and even skeptical. We are the underdogs, and to emerge victorious will take so much time that it's likely many of us will not live to see the changes we know are due.

Which makes the so-called little issues that much more important. You can swear off McDonald's and Pepsi—iconic brands, but not the only ones worth boycotting—right now. Most of you can begin to cook. You can teach your youngest kid to eat better than your oldest. You can garden, or grow parsley on your windowsill. You can cook your favorite dish for your kid's classroom, or get your kid to cook his or her favorite dish with you. You can force yourself and your loved ones to eat a salad every Monday, or Wednesday for that matter. You can probably pay a little more for food and support a farmer who isn't growing a thousand acres of corn. You can eat an apple instead of a cookie. For breakfast, you can eat leftovers of something you made for dinner.

These are not always easy things to do. Like New Year's resolutions, they may have to be addressed time and again. If you once stopped smoking or once started exercising, or did anything else that was challenging, you probably recognize two things: One, changing your relationship to food is a difficult thing. Two, it can be done.

I recognize that this is preachy. There is something about the nature of becoming public—of listening and speaking instead of writing—that demands a direct response. It feels immodest and perhaps it is. But I'm encountering hundreds of people every day, and the ones I speak to individually usually say one of two things: "You've helped me change my life," or "Please help me figure out how to change my life." The answers are already out there; it's all been said already, by me and dozens of other people: The small things, the seemingly little changes, they do matter.

"How do we change the food system?" is a question that cannot be directly answered. We elect representatives who understand what's wrong. We petition. We make noise. We don't settle for the grudging, halting, sometimes downright stupid changes that government agencies make, but demand more. We don't know the end but we push for progress. We don't quit.

But "How do I change my relationship to food?" is a question you can answer yourself, now, in a continuing manner. We need both questions. But in a way the second one, the littler one, is much more powerful.

OCTOBER 14, 2014

Acknowledgments

In this book is some of the best work I've ever done, and it's largely thanks to the generosity of others. The synthesis of thoughts is generally my own, but the stuff of those thoughts comes from elsewhere. Much of that is in print, but a great deal of it comes from conversation. It's the people I talk with and work with that really informs my columns.

I will inevitably miss some people here, because in the course of a given week I probably speak with a dozen people about my column, some more formally than others. But in general they fall into three groups, those inside the *New York Times* (or formerly so); those in the food, academic, agricultural, government, and other worlds; and those in my personal life.

Thanks to all of you.

At the *Times*: Lawrence Downes, Andy Rosenthal, David Shipley, George Kalogerakis, Bill Keller, Chris Conway, Rick Berke, Laura Chang, Erika Goode, Sewell Chang, Roberta Zeff, Honor Jones, John Guida, Jennifer Mascia, Lydia Dallett, and especially Trish Hall and Kelly Doe.

In the world at large: This is impossible, really—there are a thousand people to thank here. But I've been guided and advised most by Ricardo Salvador, Michael Pollan, and Marion Nestle. Also super-helpful over the years have been David Ludwig, Gary Taubes, Laura Rogers, Jenny Powers, Wendell Berry, Mark Arax, Bill Niman, Chellie Pingree, Paul Shapiro, Raj Patel, Mike Licht. There are more, a thousand more . . .

In my "real" life: Pam Krauss, Angela Miller, Trish Hall, Kate Bittman, Emma Baar-Bittman, Gertrude Bittman, and Kelly Doe.

—MARK BITTMAN
NEW YORK, JANUARY 2015

Index